THE
CNA
TRAINING
SOLUTION

Trainer's Manual

SECOND EDITION

Kelly Smith Papa, RN, BSN
Judith Ryan, RN, BSN

The CNA Training Solution: Trainer's Manual, Second Edition is published by HCPro, Inc.

Kelly Smith Papa, RN, BSN, Contributing Editor
Judith Ryan, RN, BSN, Contributing Editor
Elizabeth Petersen, Executive Editor
Sada Preisch, Proofreader
Mike Mirabello, Senior Graphic Artist

Brian Babineau, Layout Artist
Jean St. Pierre, Director of Operations
Patrick Campagnone, Cover Designer
Emily Sheahan, Group Publisher

Advice given is general. Readers should consult professional counsel for specific legal, ethical, or clinical questions.

Arrangements can be made for quantity discounts. For more information, contact:

HCPro, Inc.
P.O. Box 1168
Marblehead, MA 01945
Telephone: 800/650-6787 or 781/639-1872
Fax: 781/639-2982
E-mail: *customerservice@hcpro.com*

Visit HCPro at its World Wide Web sites:
www.hcpro.com and *www.hcmarketplace.com*

Contents

         The CNA Training Solution: Trainer's Manual, Second Edition

ABOUT THE CONTRIBUTING EDITORS

Kelly Smith Papa, RN, BSN

Kelly Smith Papa, RN, BSN, is the clinical educator at the McLean Nursing Facility in Connecticut. Prior to her current position, Smith Papa served as director of nursing services and as an MDS and resident care coordinator. She leads the educational needs of her facility's 600 staff members and has also been instrumental in developing seminars for healthcare professionals in her community. Smith Papa also currently serves as the senior advisor for the **Long-Term Care Nursing Advisor** e-mail newsletter and is the author of the *Inservice Training Guide: Strategies for Effective Long-Term Care Staff Education*, both published by HCPro, Inc.

Judith Ryan, RN, BSN

Judith Ryan, RN, BSN, has more than 20 years of nursing experience and is currently director of staff development at Abbott House nursing home in Massachusetts. Ryan is responsible for the training and educational programs for the facility's entire staff. She also currently serves as the senior advisor for **CNA Training Advisor,** a monthly inservice newsletter published by HCPro, Inc.

INTRODUCTION

"THE JOB OF AN EDUCATOR IS TO TEACH STUDENTS TO SEE THE VITALITY IN THEMSELVES."

–Joseph Campbell, mythologist and educator

A good teacher is an inspiration. Whether it's a parent, an older sibling, neighbor, friend, or classroom instructor, you never forget the lessons taught by a good teacher. The best teachers awaken something inside that makes you want to learn.

As a staff educator, your role is both important and challenging. You are faced with training CNAs and nurses who are busy and sometimes unresponsive to traditional inservices. That's where this training kit comes in. You now have every tool you'll need to make your inservice education program a success. Inside you'll find creative methods for making inservices fun and interesting, as well as educational.

From games to activities to facility-wide events to the interactive *Caregiver's Workbook*, we've provided everything you need to craft an effective training program for your entire frontline staff. Our goal was to make it easier for you to excel as the kind of teacher who inspires as well as educates. The next step is up to you.

Good luck and have fun!

CHAPTER 1

Facility policy and procedure training

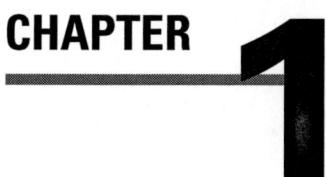

FACILITY POLICY AND PROCEDURE TRAINING

While you train staff members with the inservices in this book, keep in mind the additional information they will need to know regarding your facility's specific policies and procedures. It is your responsibility to ensure that staff members learn your facility's policies and procedures that impact their jobs.

Review the necessary manuals to get a general idea of the requirements for your facility's education and training policies and procedures. Procedural modifications to this trainer's manual will have to be made locally. These modifications include incorporating training on your facility's procedures into your overall education and training plan.

This additional training can be accomplished in a variety of ways, including:

- Incorporating the facility's policies and procedures appropriately into inservices

- Hands-on training such as role playing

- Policy and procedures handbooks (or think of another creative way of providing the training; this manual may give you some ideas)

CHAPTER 2

How these training tools work

CHAPTER 2

How these training tools work

In order to keep staff up to date about clinical and care topics they'll need to do their jobs properly, you will need to cover a great deal of information in your training sessions. For truly effective training, incorporate discussions of real-world applications of care techniques by using case examples and by allowing learners to come up with and share answers to their own case examples. But when the ideal length for a stand-alone inservice is typically 30–45 minutes and inservices should never be longer than one hour, how can you accomplish all of this and still control the amount of time your staff will need to devote to training sessions?

Planning your education training sessions

Consider various ways of conducting your education and training sessions to determine which will best achieve your objectives. Regardless of which option you choose, take into account the following suggestions:

- If you choose to conduct your inservices in a classroom setting and focus exclusively on material covered in the *Caregiver's Workbook*, be sure to check the staff's understanding by stopping your presentation at least three or four times for questions. Spend five minutes providing a case scenario to communicate the real-world application of the material.

- Begin every inservice with an overview of your objectives (located, in this manual, at the beginning of each lesson) to specify what learners should accomplish both during and after the sessions.

- If you plan to hold on to staff workbooks, make sure that learners know where to find them so they can refer to their workbooks when necessary. Store the workbooks in an accessible location. For easy reference and to have staff take ownership of their training, have each person fill in his or her name with a marker on the space allotted on the workbooks' cover.

- Provide learners with a follow-up contact person and a mechanism for asking questions. Following an inservice, questions may arise and learners need to know that they are always welcome to ask them.

- Throughout the year, conduct refresher presentations and reiterate important information through fairs, posters, videos, or case-scenario questions posed in facility newsletters.

Review Chapter 3 in this manual for more on training methods you can use to ensure that learners understand and apply the information you teach in each inservice.

The material you choose to include in each inservice will likely depend on the size of your group. In addition, different staff members have different responsibilities, so modify each session to match the participants' roles and needs. The learner handout tools in this manual have been developed specifically to allow you to modify and customize them as appropriate.

Using the training tools

Once you decide how to approach staff training, you will need to know how to use the training tools, such as this manual, the *Caregiver's Workbook*, and the *Training Treasure Chest* CD-ROM. Each is designed to help you train CNAs on the topics specific to their jobs. When combined, these training tools will help you give staff optimal training with the least amount of footwork for you:

1. ***Trainer's Manual.*** This manual has 11 chapters, and includes the following:

   - **Lesson plans.** The lessons within the *Trainer's Manual* include specific directions and talking points for you, the staff development trainer. The directions include a brief overview of what you will be teaching staff, how long the inservice should take, what materials you will need to prepare for the session, and how the inservice is intended to be taught.

   - **Instruction icons.** Throughout the trainer's inservices, you will find icons that cue you to initiate discussions or perform activities or inform you that a certain piece of text is only in the *Trainer's Manual* and not in the *Caregiver's Workbook*. (See p. 10 for different icons and their definitions.)

   - **Activities.** Each inservice includes activities with instructions. Some are listed only in the *Trainer's Manual*, but most can be found in both the manual and the *Caregiver's Workbook*. The adaptable games in Chapter 4 are not found within the workbook but are included in this manual to keep training fun and interesting.

2. *Caregiver's Workbook.* Each staff member receives a *Caregiver's Workbook* that consists of the 10 lessons to be taught in combination with the *Trainer's Manual.* Each lesson includes written activities, care tips, compassion tips, and more, all of which are also found in the *Trainer's Manual.*

3. *Training Treasure Chest.* The *Training Treasure Chest* is a CD-ROM that provides you with a creative way to reinforce inservice education and training. It contains quizzes, handouts to accompany each inservice, certificates of completion, sample education and training games and contests, and other training tools to make inservices fun, effective, and, best of all, interactive:

- **Handouts.** The handouts should be used in conjunction with the inservice. Handouts will generally provide interesting facts or key information to underline the issues covered in the inservice. Handouts are only found on the CD-ROM and must be printed prior to the session.

- **Quizzes.** Each inservice comes with an accompanying quiz. Use the quizzes to test staff comprehension of the lesson and to document mandatory training. The quizzes are not in the *Caregiver's Workbook* and therefore must be printed prior to each inservice session. However, they are found in this manual and on the CD-ROM within the folder for each inservice topic. Quizzes are completely customizable, so feel free to add or delete questions for your training.

- **Certificates of completion.** Awarding certificates of completion to CNAs shows that you care about their professional development. Following each quiz, hand out certificates of completion to each staff member who scores a 70% or higher. The certificates of completion can be found in this manual and on the CD-ROM. They can be modified to suit your facility's needs.

Instruction icons

The following icons will cue you through each inservice:

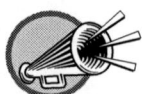 **Trainer talking tip:** This icon shows when you need to talk or read instructions.

 **Instruction icon:** This icon lets you know when you must do something within the inservice (e.g., pass out a handout, etc).

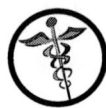 **Caregiving tip:** The caregiving icon helps caregivers quickly find important information regarding resident care.

 **Compassion tip:** This icon highlights advice or "things to remember" for caregivers.

 **Just-for-trainers tip:** This icon marks important information that can only be found in the *Trainer's Manual*. This information is not in the *Caregiver's Workbook*; it is up to you to share it with learners.

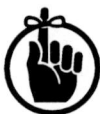 **Reminder tip:** This icon highlights important facts or tips that caregivers must remember when doing their jobs.

The Training Treasure Chest *CD-ROM contents*

The CD-ROM includes:

Instructor aids

- Sample inservice calendar
- Sample inservice poster
- Sample training reminder note
- Sample training documentation log
- Form A: Rate the trainer learner evaluation form
- Form B: Rate the training learner evaluation form
- Helpful links

Games

- Caregiver Pursuit sample category, question, and answer cards
- Out of Jeopardy sample answers and questions
- Facility-Family Feud sample questions and answers

Tools

- Sample flashcards
- Sample cheat sheet

Inservice folders

Quizzes and certificates of completion for all lessons are located within inservice folders.

Documentation

- While facility policies differ on what and how CNAs can document, it's important to train your CNAs to recognize and report problems and changes in condition.

- CNAs often spend more time with our residents than virtually any other staff member, and they usually are the first to notice declines in health or other issues.

To help with CNA documentation and reporting, we've provided you with the following forms and tools:

- CNA weekly skin assessment
- ADL flowsheet
- Nursing assistant cleaning schedule
- Seven-day resident self ability evaluation
- Nursing assistant assignment sheet
- Vital sign flow record
- ADL/restorative nursing flowsheet
- Cognitive/mood/behavioral data collection flowsheet

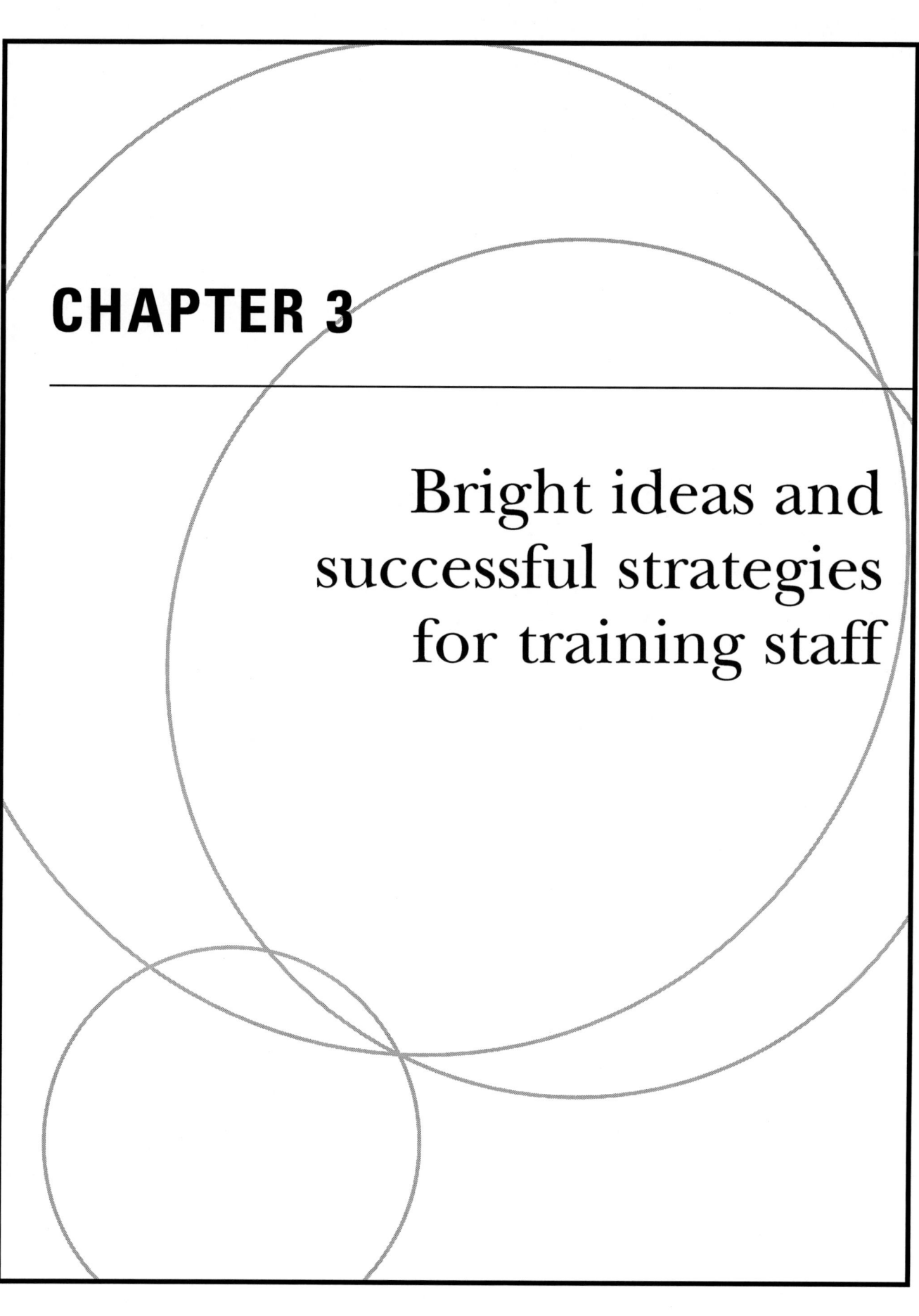

CHAPTER 3

Bright ideas and successful strategies for training staff

CHAPTER 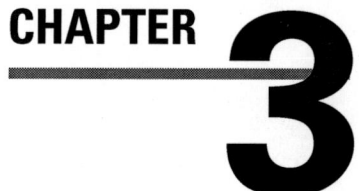 3

BRIGHT IDEAS AND SUCCESSFUL STRATEGIES FOR TRAINING STAFF

Overview

Each state requires that certified nursing assistants (CNAs) receive a certain number of training hours per year to remain certified and to continue giving care. You are therefore required to offer regular education and training to CNAs so they can earn their mandatory training hours.

All CNAs need to be trained on the same topics, but because all individuals learn differently, you should use a variety of teaching mechanisms to accomplish the task.

This section provides examples of such mechanisms. It also provides information to help prepare and develop inservice education and training. It will cover:

- What training is required

- Fundamentals of training—your goals in the inservice session

- Education and training techniques (e.g., approaches to adult education, creative ideas for effective education and training, and ways to monitor awareness and understanding)

- Techniques to follow up the education and training

What training is required

As previously mentioned, the number of training hours CNAs must have depends on the state in which they work and generally spans from 12–24 hours annually.

Within those hours, you are required to teach certain inservices each year in order to comply with facility, state, federal, OSHA, and Joint Commission (or any other accreditation association) requirements. The mandatory inservice topics typically include abuse and neglect prevention, Resident's Rights, the

Health Insurance Portability and Accountability Act of 1996 (HIPAA), infection control, pain management, and age-specific care. Beyond mandatory topics, the training must also include areas of physical care, communication, and psychosocial issues. As the staff development coordinator, you have a plethora of interesting care topics from which to choose.

Once you research which inservices are required (and by which entities), be sure to include them in your inservice calendar for the year. When preparing such calendars for staff and advertising inservices, make sure that you indicate those that are mandatory.

You will need to retrain staff if your facility changes any of its policies and procedures. Therefore, someone must be in charge of monitoring the policies and procedures and alerting the trainer when new training is required.

State- and facility-specific policies and procedures

Individual states and facilities have their own policies and procedures for particular topics, and you need to educate staff on them. These topics often include Resident's Rights, infection control, and abuse and neglect prevention. When preparing and teaching such inservices, insert and explain any and all policies and procedures that are specific to your facility and state. Print copies and show learners how your facility's or state's regulations are different from those of the federal government—doing so shows staff that you take care and respect for residents very seriously and that you expect a high level of care for residents.

Your audience

You will need to train your facility's entire staff, which may include anyone from CNAs to clergy. Your audience, therefore, will vary constantly, so be aware of the obstacles you will likely encounter when trying to meet the training needs for all of your staff. For instance, when teaching staff about HIPAA, give them tips that are specific to their jobs to help them protect and preserve privacy and confidentiality. People must relate to information in order to comprehend and retain it. When giving staff care or other tips, make sure that they can apply them directly to their jobs.

Fundamentals of training—your goals in the inservice session

Do you have an extensive background in training, or is this your first time training? Have you attended seminars that have helped you hone training skills, or have you done your best and had to "wing it"?

We have all certainly found ourselves in some sort of formalized learning setting as adults. You can probably think of good and bad examples of previous trainings. What do the good examples have in common? What do the bad examples have in common?

Often, the good and the bad examples have the trainer as a common denominator: Successful training depends upon the skill of the trainer. You can be a successful trainer whether or not you have spent years practicing to be a trainer or attending multiple train-the-trainer courses. Confidence in yourself as the trainer, trust in the learners to learn, and interactive, discovery-led learning are the key skills for leading a successful training session.

Become a successful trainer

Experienced trainers across the board say the most important accessory they can wear is an air of confidence. If you are sure of your skills and well prepared for the training (in terms of both the material and the human factor), you can approach the training session confidently and handle any situation.

Assess your skills

If you have previously conducted training sessions, then you have a great library of experience to review. Even if this is your first time training, though, you have very likely been in a situation where you have had to teach or convey information. Keep these situations in mind, and try the following exercise to inventory your skills and determine your strengths.

Exercise 1: Inventory your skills and determine your strengths

1. How do you work with others? Do you tend to take charge, or do you prefer to let others lead?

2. How are you smart? Is it your analytical, creative, or practical intelligence that is the strongest?

3. How do you communicate? When you explain something, do you ask your listeners if they understand what you are saying? Do your listeners tend to follow easily what you are saying? While speaking, are you aware of your listeners' reactions?

4. Do you consider yourself more introverted or more extroverted?

Regardless of your answers, you have strength in each of the above areas. Capitalizing on your strengths and incorporating them into your training will help you conduct a successful training session. But just how do you do that?

Examples of ways to use your strengths

1. **Working with others**

   If you answered, "I prefer to let others take charge," then you do not consider yourself assertive when working with others. You might think that this is a weakness for a trainer, but it can actually be a strength. One of the best ways adults can learn is by discovering the answers themselves. Consider training by letting your learners take charge in the training session.

   If you answered, "I definitely take charge," then you are in a good position to guide the learners through the training goals. However, although being assertive is a strength for a training session, being aggressive is not. Consider also using interactive elements in your training sessions, such as question-and-answer sessions or games.

   Get to know your learners because they too will have varying answers to the above questions. You may need to modify your technique somewhat in order to best respond to your learners' needs.

2. **Your intelligence**

   By basic definition, intelligence is the ability to achieve goals. Each of us has the ability to be analytical, creative, and practical, but you probably feel that you are stronger in one or another of these areas. All three areas are important, but most important is achieving a balance and employing your strongest area to its utmost.

   For example, if you consider yourself primarily analytical, you should be able to review the inservice material, spot patterns in the information, compare and contrast information, and thoroughly instruct your learners. If you consider yourself more practical, you should be able to review the inservice material and then spot ways in which it affects each staff member and how it impacts real-life, day-to-day work. If you consider yourself more creative, you should be able to review the inservice material and think of fun and interesting ways to present the information.

   Consider that your learners will be an amalgam of these types of intelligence, which means that the way you teach may not be the way your learner learns. So how do you balance these intelligences and achieve learning? Consider letting your learners interact in a way that uses their type of intelligence (for example, a question-and-answer session can allow learners to ask the types of questions that help them learn), and let the learners' strengths balance yours (for example, a practical learner might spot a real-world application of a point you are teaching). The best solution is to build a training session that presents the information using a variety of methods, such as lectures, question-and-answer sessions, and games.

3. **Your communication skills**

   Your presentation skills, which include both speaking and listening, are among the most important elements of your ability to successfully train others. First, keep your message succinct and relevant. Use effective communication techniques, such as making sure that your learners understand what you are saying; tuning in to your learners' nonverbal clues, such as body language, to understand how they are reacting and if they are following what you are saying; keeping in mind your role in the interaction (i.e., source of information rather than keeper of order); making eye contact with your learners; and letting the session be a dialogue—encouraging interaction and participation—by both encouraging and asking questions. In short, pay attention to communication, notice your learners' reactions, and involve voices other than your own.

4. **Your interactive personality**

   Carl Jung broadly discussed personality types, including the two differing and opposing attitudes: extroversion and introversion. We've all heard that extroverts like to be sociable and prefer being with groups of people, and that introverts, while able to socialize and enjoy it, prefer to be alone and ultimately find socializing draining. How does being more of one type or the other impact your ability to train?

The theory is that these attitudes affect your method of speech. In general, extroverts often think as they speak. Introverts often think and then speak. One is not better than the other; rather, each has its own strength. If you can form ideas while interacting with others, then you may be better at altering the training while it's in process to best address learner needs. If you reflect and form ideas internally and then speak, then you may be better at addressing learner questions and concerns accurately. Find your strengths and gear the training to take advantage of them.

Knowing who you are—knowing and believing in your strengths—is the first step toward creating a situation in which you can succeed and be confident. Preparing for training is, in large part, preparing yourself. Take the time to further consider your personality and strengths, including what you think of yourself and what others think of you, and ponder how you might use these to best address questions and issues that arise during training. Anticipating situations and knowing how you will address them—and believing in your ability to do so well—will accomplish the major goal of all trainers: project an image of confidence.

Identify disruptive learners

You know the person in a classroom who always, somehow, disrupts the learning flow? Is there one in every class? How do you handle that situation? Can you prevent it?

Conventional wisdom holds that most disruptive learners are bored, nervous, or insecure in the learning environment for some reason. If you understand the likely reason why, then you can take steps to prevent problems. If that doesn't work, then there are some good methods to employ to address the problem.

The bored or uninterested learner

This learner probably does not know why he or she is in training or how the material is relevant, much less how it is essential. This learner may also not be receiving information in a way that is congruent with his or her learning style.

The debater learner

This learner expresses critical, disagreeing, or disapproving opinions about the material or your facility's policies. The debater learner may also use the training session to vent disagreement with other facility policies or events. The most dangerous kind of debater learner, however, is one who is frustrated by the way the training will affect his or her job and takes out that frustration on the trainer, fellow learners, or material in general. A bad attitude toward information is contagious. As the leader in the situation, you will need to moderate interaction. Be careful to not let an assertive or aggressive learner take over the training session, and be careful to not penalize the entire class for the actions of one learner.

The joker learner

This learner perpetually makes jokes or maintains a running, humorous commentary during the training. The jokes may or may not be relevant to the material. Humor is a good way to learn, and the on-topic jokes may be a way for you to engage this learner and help him or her retain the lessons. However, this learner may become disruptive if the jokes are too frequent or off-topic. Also note that the jokes may also be a sign of boredom or disinterest.

The late-arrival learner

Whether it's intentional or not, some learners may arrive after training has already begun. A late arrival, as discreet as the person may attempt to be when entering, shifts the learners' focus away from you and from the material. This disruption is the easiest type to resolve. Offer a simple greeting ("Hello, welcome.") and immediately resume presenting the material where you left off. Do not recap the material for the late arrival, demand an explanation for the tardiness, or in any other way extend the disruption.

The questioner learner (a.k.a. the interrupter)

Although question-and-answer is an excellent technique for successful training, questions have their time and place in the training presentation. Some learners may leap ahead to a concept you have yet to present, interrupting the flow with a comment or question. Others may frequently interrupt with critiques of plans or policies. Regardless of the type of interruption, it can become disruptive to the session. Because your presentation has a logical order, stay on track as best you can. Be careful how you solve this disruption because you do not want to discourage questions or cause learners to keep confusion or concern to themselves.

The "I don't get it" learner

Your learners will enter the classroom with many long-held beliefs about teaching and learning. You can't know all of their backgrounds, but assume that at least several of them have had negative learning experiences or a negative view of their ability to learn. If one of your learners has a "learning block" and your attempts to use different methods of explaining a concept or different training techniques fail, then you may need to address it in another way and at another time.

Handle disruptive learners

What do these learners have in common? They are all disengaged from learning and pose the potential risk of disengaging other learners as well. Therefore, create a vested, cognitive interest in the learning for all learners. Following are a few suggestions:

- Set training goals for the course and share them with learners

- Communicate to learners how the material is relevant to them and why they are in the training class

- Involve the learners (e.g., use games)

- Use a variety of teaching styles

- Monitor learning and understanding (e.g., ask questions and pay attention to body language to make sure that your learners are still engaged in learning)

If, despite attempts to prevent problems, you determine that some of the learners are disengaged from learning, then you will need to solve the problem. Following are a few suggestions about how to do that:

- Maintain your role as moderator; do not become the authority figure. For example, if the problem is the debater learner, try to find out why the learner is being disruptive. You may learn that the person is worried about his or her job and how the information will impact it. Perhaps this person is worried he or she will not remember what you're teaching. If the person is simply disgruntled, let that person know that although you understand his or her concerns, you and the other learners can't effect change in the training session. Gently remind the learners of the purpose and goals of the session, and encourage the debater learner to address concerns with his or her manager. Validation is important, as is keeping yourself in your role (as moderator/trainer) and on track (focus on the purpose and goals of the training).

- Acknowledge the behavior. For example, if you have a joker learner, acknowledge the humor but keep it in line and prevent it from distracting from the material and schedule by quickly moving on to the next point. If the joker persists and becomes too much of an interruption, perhaps you can respond with humor, and let the learners and jokers know that at the conclusion of the course, you will make time for questions, answers, and jokes, too.

- Accept your fallibility. For example, if the problem is bored learner(s), acknowledge that your presentation may have gotten too dry, you may have lectured too long, or, in some way, the learners have become disengaged. Your best solution is to change the pace (i.e., speed it up or slow it down, as needed) and try another training technique.

- Try to change the method of explanation or the training technique. For example, if, during a lecture portion of the training presentation you get an "I don't get it" learner, try switching to another technique, such as question-and-answer. Perhaps by listening to questions from others, this learner will grasp the concept, or at least feel less anxious about not understanding a point.

- Suggest more productive ways for the learner to participate, while offering assurance that the problem will be addressed. For example, if the problem is a questioner or interrupter learner, suggest that all learners write down questions as they occur to them; assure all learners that if the material does not cover that point of concern or confusion, you will set aside time specifically for questions and answers. Promise that all questions will get answered eventually.

- Keep on track. Doing so is the most important response to any of the disruptions.

Mix and match any of these problem-solving techniques, or move through them in a sort of progressive order.

Most important, in handling any problem learner, do not let your response become emotional, become more of a disruption, break your bond with the other learners, or disengage the other learners. Let the disruption become a learning opportunity. At the very least, you will have gained insight into one of your learners, and it may help you acquire a good technique to employ or give you a good candidate for a specific role in a game. Even challenges can become golden opportunities.

Understanding and insight are the keys that unlock the problem and provide the solution. Once you understand why the problem is occurring, you are in a better position to address it. But be careful not to lose too much time addressing one person's problem and get too far away from the material and schedule. Focusing too much on one learner is a sure way to disengage other learners and create more problems.

Exercise 2: Address sample problems

Situation 1: You have just finished detailing ways to properly defuse outbursts from residents suffering from Alzheimer's disease. During your presentation, one learner, Marcy, constantly asked whether certain techniques she came across in her job as a nurse's aide were appropriate for calming aggravated residents with the disease. You answered each question. You have now moved on to the next part of the presentation and are discussing the different ways to care for residents who wander. Marcy continues to interject questions about particular experiences with the resident outbursts and how she should have handled them. What kind of learner is Marcy, what can you deduce about why she is still asking questions, and how might you handle the situation?

Things to consider: Very likely, Marcy is a combination of the "I don't get it" learner and the questioner learner. Considering Marcy's job, what elements of the training might be more important to her than others? Might those be the same priorities of others in the class?

Suggestions: Marcy is clearly missing the next part of your presentation because she is still focused on the previous topic. Further, she is steering you off track and preventing the other learners from learning the information. At this time, pause in the training and ask the class, not Marcy specifically, whether they need to review the last segment of training. If the majority says no, prepare to move forward. However, validate the needs of those who say yes, and assure them that they can ask more questions during the question-and-answer segment of the training class. Suggest that they write down questions as they come up. Also, remind them that you or another appropriate expert will be available to answer day-to-day/course-work questions after training is complete.

If the majority says yes, then review the points in the last segment. Do not present the information in exactly the same way; try a different technique, and maybe incorporate a game. Knowledge Bowl is an easy game to play and is explained in Chapter 4 of this manual. Consider pairing learners and have each take a turn teaching the other about problem concepts.

Situation 2: A staff member enters the training session late. You have just concluded the greetings, but have yet to move on to the main presentation. This staff member selects a chair as far from the front of the room as possible. Then, during the course of training, she frequently makes comments to her neighbors, who seem uncomfortable. By the middle of the training, she has begun to get louder and louder with her criticisms, such as "That's ridiculous! How do they expect us to do our jobs with that constraint?"

Things to consider: Very likely, this staff member is a combination of the late arrival and the debater. Unfortunately, because she was late, you do not know this woman's name, nor do you know her position. However, you can see that she is frustrated. Is she having a bad day? Or is she really this frustrated with the information you're teaching in the lesson?

Suggestions: At this point, the disruptions may have caused other learners to disengage from the learning. A few have begun interrupting with concerns generated from comments the debater learner has made. Pause the training. Using "I" statements rather than "you" statements, first acknowledge the behavior, perhaps by saying, "I notice that some of this material concerns you." Ask her why she is concerned and find out her name and job. Finally, remind her that the purpose of the training session simply is to convey information rather than to effect change. Suggest a more appropriate time and place to pursue her concerns.

Note: It is helpful to know the learners in advance of the training session. If possible, get information for each such as name, job title, and reporting manager.

Situation 3: You look around the room and find that very few learners are looking at you. You aren't getting good eye contact.

Things to consider: Your learners do not seem engaged or interested. Many of them are likely bored or disinterested learners. Who is in your class? What technique were you using and what information were you discussing when you last were aware of holding their interest?

Suggestions: Review the information you are currently presenting using another training technique.

Feedback and learning retention

One of the best ways to refine your techniques and be the best trainer possible is to get feedback from your learners.

Training techniques: How to train adult learners

It is important that you know the audience you are training. When getting to know your audience, consider their:

- Jobs and responsibilities

- Goals in the training

- Potential knowledge of the material

- Age (i.e., not numerical, but the fact that they are adults)

Some of your learners may already know quite a bit about the information you are presenting. Some may know nothing at all. Although your learners may have very little in common, they do share one characteristic: They are all adults. They have special requirements when it comes to learning, and thus you should use methods of training that are more effective for adults.

Learning styles of adults

Did you know there is a specific word for adult learning? "Andragogy," a term coined by Malcolm Knowles, is the art and science of helping adults learn. Knowles was a leading expert in the adult education field. Greg Kearsley, a specialist of adult education and technology, says the existence of andragogy "means that instruction for adults needs to focus more on the process and less on the content being taught. Strategies such as case studies, role playing, simulations, and self-evaluations are most useful. Instructors adopt a role of facilitator or resource rather than lecturer or grader".[1]

James Atherton, a principal lecturer on education, elaborates on Kearsley's statement and explains the five elements of adult learning:

- **The need to know**—Adult learners are problem centered. They need to know why they should learn something before they begin to learn it.

- **Learner self-concept**—Adults need to be responsible for their own decisions and need to be treated as capable of self-direction.

- **Role of learners' experience**—Adult learners have a variety of experiences of life, which form the richest resource for learning. These experiences, however, are saturated with bias and presupposition.

- **Readiness to learn**—Adults are ready to learn whatever they need to know in order to cope effectively with life situations.

- **Orientation to learning**—Adults are motivated to learn to the extent that they perceive the material's ability to help them perform tasks they confront in their life situations.

For adult learners, the process of training is more important than the content. Consider using techniques that achieve the adult learner's goal in learning.[2]

Set trainer teaching and learner learning goals

You know your specific task in conducting the inservice, and learners are generally compelled to attend. But how do you engage the learners? The very first thing you need to do is establish goals.

State the need for training, relate it as closely as possible to each learner in the class, and have each learner state his or her learning goals. Give an overview of the information you are going to present. Consider preparing learners for any special or creative techniques you will use to present the information.

Emphasize the need to know

People rarely exert effort for or freely contribute time to something that holds no interest or relevance to them. Adult learners especially need to know why they should learn what you are teaching. Therefore, let the learners understand the "problem" as it relates to them and help to solve it. Play a training game or have all of them cite examples from their jobs that are relevant to the training. Facility-family Feud is a good game to help learners think of how the training information is relevant to them. This game is explained in Chapter 4 of this manual.

Treat the adult learners . . . like adults

Although there is a distinction between the roles of learner and teacher, the best teachers are mentors. That statement relies on the connotation of the word "mentor," so to be clearer, consider this:

The definition of mentor is "trusted counselor or guide," and its synonyms include coach and tutor. Therefore, a mentor implies a relationship of equals, one of whom is sharing or imparting knowledge and experience in an adult-to-adult interaction.

Thus, for adults in a training class, you will achieve your best success when you act as a mentor and facilitator and let the adult learners be responsible for their own decisions. Treat them as capable of self-direction, and your learners will live up to your belief in them.

Pacing

Pace the presentation of the material to your learners' knowledge and interest level. For instance, imagine teaching an inservice about confidentiality and the rules of HIPAA. Some learners, such as clergy, may wish to spend more time discussing how to handle questions from friends and family members of the patient that may infringe on privacy. Other learners, such as medical work force, may wish to focus on hallway conversations and how they might infringe on privacy policies. If you have a mixed group with varying interests, make sure not to spend too much time on one issue or one specific group of learners.

Methods to increase learning retention

One of your most important objectives in training is to ensure that your learners retain what they learn. Keep in mind that people have different learning styles; therefore, you should consider using a variety of activities in your training. There are some tried-and-true methods that will promote learning retention.

1. **Apply what is learned.**
    - Provide real-life scenarios and ask the learners to comply with the facility's privacy policies and procedures.
    - Ask learners to make up the scenarios or suggest situations they've experienced.

2. **Let the learner be the trainer.**
    - Divide learners into teams and play Caregiver Pursuit. (See Chapter 4.)
    - Pair learners with quiz flashcards and have partners alternate quizzing each other.

3. **Prevent boredom.**
    - Use games, events, and rewards.
    - Use tools such as flashcards and cheat sheets.

Encourage inservice attendance

The most important thing you can do as a trainer is remember your audience. Think about the staff you'll be training and try to appeal to them when advertising for your inservices. For instance, if you know that certain caregivers like to get their information by playing games, advertise that you'll be playing Caregiver Pursuit or another game that will hold their attention.

Respect the accumulated life experience

Most of your learners have likely been around at least one block. The accumulated experience they bring with them into the training session will affect how they learn, how they interact, what is important to them, and so on. Keep this in mind as you train, and always pay attention to the reactions of your learners.

Keep it real

Create practical and real-life situations in which your learners share their experiences and then apply the information you're teaching to those situations. Ask each learner to provide an example from his or her job. As Atherton stated, "Adults are motivated to learn to the extent that they perceive that it will help them perform tasks they confront in their life situations." Keep your learners engaged by relating the material to their day-to-day tasks and how the information affects it.

Monitor awareness and understanding during training

One of the fundamental training skills is to pay close attention to your learners—make sure that they are engaged in learning and retaining the lessons. You can do so indirectly by watching body language and interpreting behavior. However, you can also monitor awareness and understanding by employing interactive training techniques, such as games, quizzes, role playing, and so on.

Use discovery and inquiry-led training

The University of Texas at Austin's College of Natural Sciences developed the Discovery Learning Project, which "promotes the development and use of discovery or inquiry-based methods of teaching and learning. This project is predicated on the belief that all learners have creative ability that can be further developed utilizing the many techniques of inquiry-based learning." This technique can be very effective in motivating adult learners, increasing participation, and improving retention. It also encourages learners to take responsibility for their learning and develop problem-solving strategies.

Lecture selectively and encourage active participation

Lecturing is the most effective way to communicate the information to staff and to acquaint them with the best ways to carry out care instructions offered within each lesson. However, in order for your learners to grasp and retain the information, balance the lecturing with active participation.

Seating

Consider how the classroom is arranged. If learners need to take notes or review handouts, ensure that they all have easy access to a desk or table. If you need the learners to interact, consider positioning seating in a manner so that all learners can see each other. This arrangement also sets up the trainer as facilitator rather than as teacher, and it may encourage learners to remain focused and interactive.

Talk individually with staff members about what you'll be addressing during the inservice. For example, if you know of specific staff members who have been struggling with a particular care or procedural topic, let them know that you are hosting an inservice on that topic and would like it if they joined you and the others. Such attention personalizes the inservice for the caregiver and helps clear up his or her questions on the topic.

FIGURE **3.1** | **SAMPLE INSERVICE POSTER**

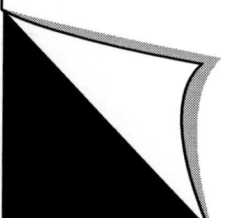

NEED A LIFT?

So do many of your residents!
Join me on Thursday, November 1, at 2 pm
or 10 pm to talk about

SAFE LIFTS, TRANSFERS & MOBILITY ASSISTS

and techniques that will save
you from back pain!

LIFT YOUR SPIRITS

And come feed your sweet tooth with the assortment
of desserts and treats that will be on display.

Please make every effort to attend
this back-saving inservice.
If you have any questions,
please call staff development.

Another way to increase inservice attendance is to advertise by putting posters in highly visible areas. Incorporate related graphics, fun fonts, borders around text, and interesting questions to grab attention as staff members pass by a bulletin board or lunchroom poster. (See Figure 3.1 for a sample inservice poster.)

Think of the inservice as a product you're trying to sell to staff members. Is it best to be aggressive and question people about why they don't show up to inservices, or is it better to give the reasons they should show up—such as games, prizes, fun, and, most important, training that helps them do their jobs better?

References

1. Kearsley, Greg. 1996. Andragogy (M. Knowles). Washington, DC: George Washington University. *http://gwis2.circ.gwu.edu:80/~kearsley/knowles.html*

2. Based on Knowles 1990: 57. Reprinted with permission. Atherton J.S. 2002. Learning and Teaching: Knowles' Andragogy [Online]: UK: Available: *www.dmu.ac.uk/~jamesa/learning/knowlesa.htm* accessed: 19 September 2002 *www.dmu.ac.uk/~jamesa/learning/knowlesa.htm*

CHAPTER 4

Games

CHAPTER 4

GAMES

Games and other activities can make training fun and interesting, and it can help your staff learn. You can adapt many popular games—including board games and quiz shows—for your education and training purposes. Although most of the games and events in this section are just fun variations on the basic question-and-answer format, variations work better with certain types of questions. For example, Caregiver Pursuit works well with questions that have only one or two correct answers, while Facility-Family Feud works well with questions that have several correct answers.

The following pages contain examples of games you can use to reinforce your education and training. Consider adapting these presentation techniques—as well as the sample hints, questions, and answers—to your facility's culture. You might also want to add your own personal flair.

Caregiver Pursuit

Based on the board game Trivial Pursuit, this game can help staff learn answers to questions about important care information presented in your inservices.

Setting up:

Create game cards using 3 x 5 index cards or pieces of construction paper; write questions on one side and their answers on the other. Organize the questions by the areas they address such as staff members, residents, symptoms, preventions, problem areas, or consequences (see Figure 4.1 for examples). Include questions that have only one or two correct answers.

How to play:

Select a group of people to question learners. As in Trivial Pursuit, each learner first chooses a category. The questioner asks the learner questions from the category of game cards until the learner answers one incorrectly, and then the questioner moves on to another learner.

Suggestion: Take advantage of this opportunity for learners to become trainers: Rotate the questioner. For example, once a learner answers incorrectly, make that learner the questioner, and rotate the former questioner into play.

Make a note of which questions learners answer correctly and which ones they answer incorrectly. Use these notes later to focus on areas that give staff the most trouble and then use the incorrectly answered questions to educate staff in future training activities.

Suggestion: Consider altering sections of the training if learners continually answer the same questions incorrectly. For example, use another training technique or emphasize the information.

Tournaments:

Create a tournament in which different classes or different departments compete against each other in order to build friendly competition and boost staff's confidence in their knowledge of the information.

FIGURE **4.1**

SAMPLE GAME: CAREGIVER PURSUIT

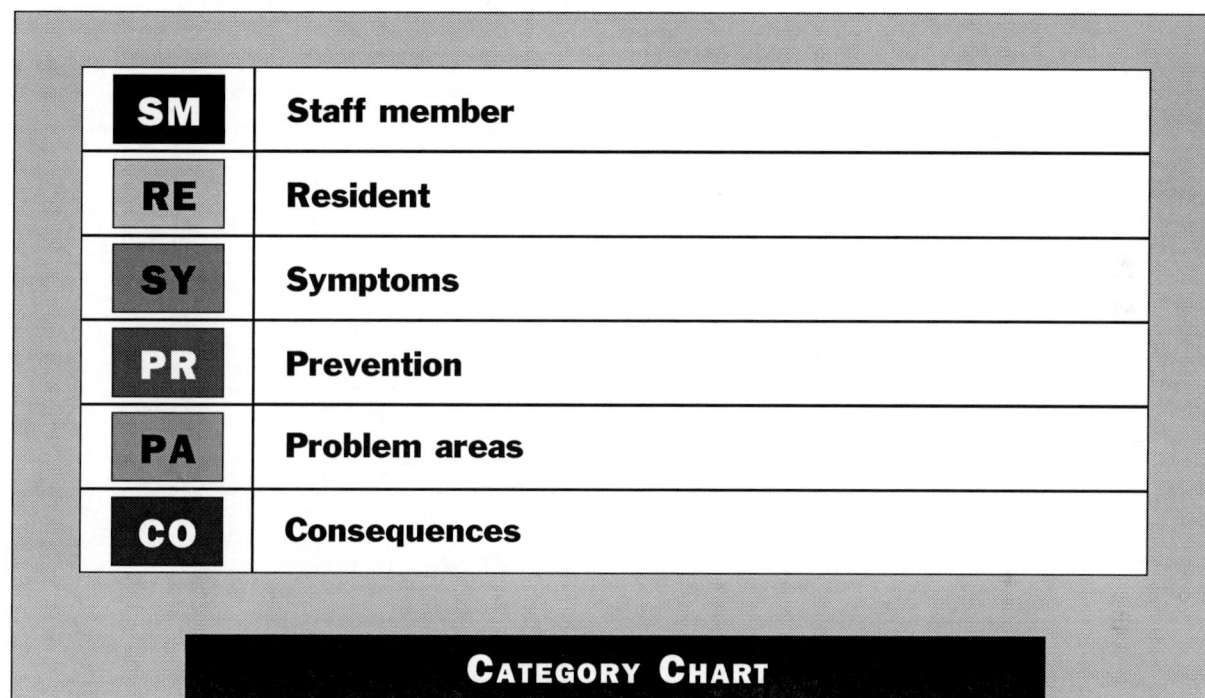

SM	Staff member
RE	Resident
SY	Symptoms
PR	Prevention
PA	Problem areas
CO	Consequences

CATEGORY CHART

 **Also appears on
your CD-ROM.**

FIGURE 4.1 | SAMPLE GAME: CAREGIVER PURSUIT (CONT.)

SKIN PROBLEMS AND CARE

Sample Questions

SM What should you do if you notice that a resident has a red pressure area that does not return to normal after 20 minutes without pressure?

RE Is it a violation of the Resident's Rights to tell a fellow caregiver about the abnormal red pressure area you discovered?

SY T/F: A skin area that is cool or cold to the touch is a symptom of a pressure sore.

PR T/F: To prevent skin problems, you should keep residents' skin clean, dry, and lubricated.

PA One of the main causes of pressure sores is constant pressure on the skin covering the _____?

CO T/F: If you don't care for frail residents' delicate skin by turning them often, and cleaning, drying, and lubricating skin with lotion, they could die from pressure sores.

Sample Answers

SM Always report your findings to the supervisor.

RE No. It is not a violation of the Resident's Rights if you inform another caregiver about a change in the resident's condition as long as he or she cares directly for the resident.

SY False. A symptom of a pressure sore is skin area that is warm or hot to the touch.

PR True.

PA Bones.

CO True. Because the frail elderly have weakened immune systems, they are much more likely to develop pressure sores and other infections they can die from.

Out of Jeopardy

Out of Jeopardy is based upon the television quiz show *Jeopardy!* Out of Jeopardy works well using both questions with one answer and those that have more than one answer. For some sample Out of Jeopardy answers and questions, see Figure 4.2. You can play Out of Jeopardy with a small or large group. You might want to have department managers play the game with their staff.

Setting up:

Write categories of answers on a chalkboard or wall. Have each column of answers be worth a certain number of points, based on the degree of difficulty of the answers in that column. Have a page of answers that correspond with the squares on the board or wall.

How to play:

Have participants, one at a time, choose questions from categories. Have the host read the answer that falls under the category and point value they've chosen, and have them guess the question. If they answer correctly, they earn the number of points the question is worth. The participant with the most points at the end of the game wins a prize. You could use different categories of questions based on the training outline, or you could create any categories you prefer.

Tournaments:

You can have an Out of Jeopardy "Tournament of Champions." One way to organize the tournament is to set it up in the cafeteria or main hallway at lunchtime so that everyone can participate. Get your administrators involved by having a member of the executive management team or governing board play the host. You could have three (or whatever number you choose) "champions" be the participants. Champions are those staff members who perform well in departmental Out of Jeopardy games or other education and training activities.

FIGURE **4.2**

SAMPLE GAME: OUT OF JEOPARDY

STANDARD PRECAUTIONS	TRANSMISSION METHODS	PPE	VACCINE	POLICIES
100 pts	100 pts	100 pts	Something all staff, residents, and visitors can do to protect residents from getting sick from influenza.	100 pts
200 pts	What happens when germs breathed through the air cause an individual to become sick.	200 pts	200 pts	200 pts
A set of rules health-care professionals must follow to protect themselves from potentially infected blood or body fluids.	300 pts	300 pts	300 pts	300 pts
400 pts	400 pts	Should be used to protect the eyes, nose, and mouth membranes from getting splashed with blood or body fluids.	400 pts	400 pts
500 pts	500 pts	500 pts	500 pts	Fill in your facility's sharps disposal policy here.

Also appears on your CD-ROM.

FIGURE 4.2

SAMPLE GAME: OUT OF JEOPARDY (CONT.)

STANDARD PRECAUTIONS	TRANSMISSION METHODS	PPE	VACCINE	POLICIES
100 pts	100 pts	100 pts	What is get the influenza (flu) vaccine?	100 pts
200 pts	What is airborne transmission?	200 pts	200 pts	200 pts
What are Standard Precautions?	300 pts	300 pts	300 pts	300 pts
400 pts	400 pts	What is a face shield?	400 pts	400 pts
500 pts	500 pts	500 pts	500 pts	What is your facility's policy regarding sharps disposal?

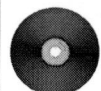 **Also appears on your CD-ROM.**

Facility-Family Feud

Facility-Family Feud is based on the television game show *Family Feud*.

Setting up:

Form two teams of staff members into different "families" to find the "top answers" to care questions. Give each team a "buzzer" (or bell) to use. You really need to brainstorm and be creative to play Facility-Family Feud. Before playing, you must come up with all the possible answers for each question.

How to play:

In Facility-Family Feud, the host (usually the trainer) asks two individuals from each team questions (see Figure 4.3 for a sample). The first person to hit his or her buzzer answers the question. If he or she gives a correct answer, his or her team will play the round. If he or she answers incorrectly then the other team gets to answer. If the opponent answers incorrectly, then the first team gets another chance. The next player in line gets to answer the original question. If the opponent answers correctly, then his or her team will play the round.

During the round, the host will ask the members of the team the same question until they get all of the answers. Write the correct answers on a chalkboard or dry-erase board as each person says them. If a team member answers incorrectly, the team gets a strike. Each team is allowed three strikes per round.

FIGURE 4.3

SAMPLE GAME: FACILITY-FAMILY FEUD

Resident's Rights

Give an example of a restraint or a possible restraint.

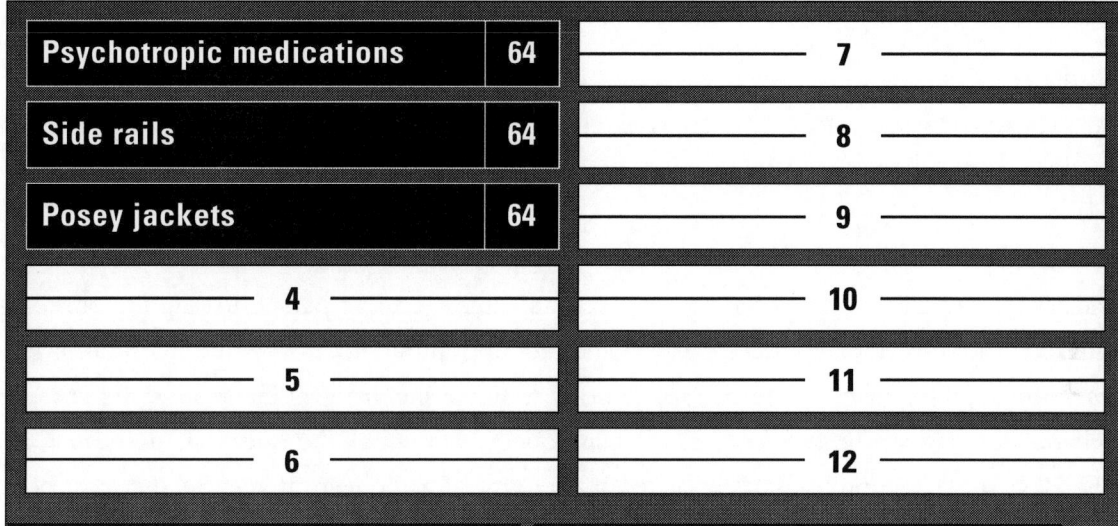

Psychotropic medications	64	7	
Side rails	64	8	
Posey jackets	64	9	
4		10	
5		11	
6		12	

Who expects you to protect the confidentiality of personal healthcare information by following the rules of the Health Insurance Portability and Accountability Act (HIPAA)?

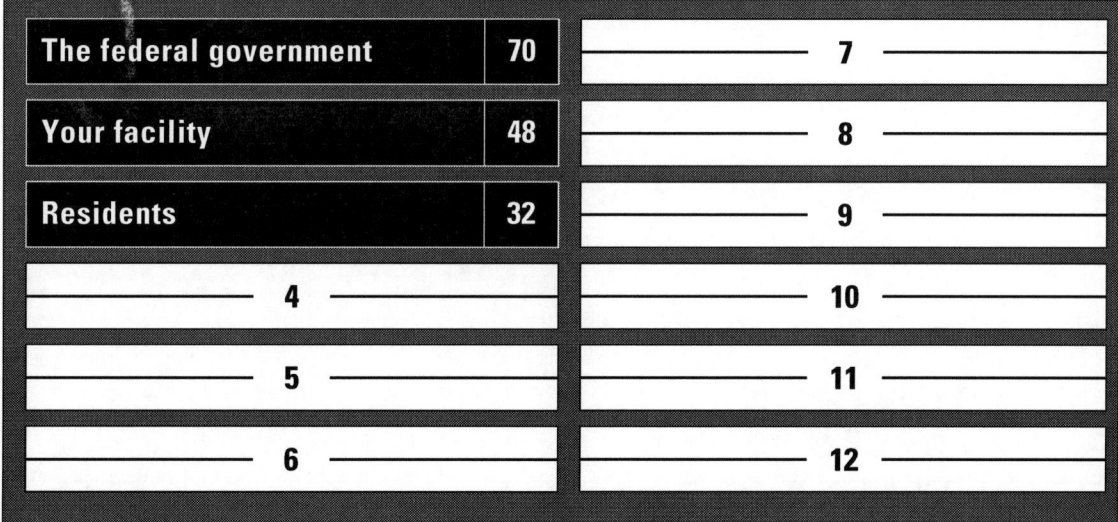

The federal government	70	7	
Your facility	48	8	
Residents	32	9	
4		10	
5		11	
6		12	

Also appears on your CD-ROM.

Knowledge Bowl

Knowledge Bowl is set up like the college bowl quiz shows seen on television. You might consider having managers play Knowledge Bowl with their departments or having two departments or work force levels challenge each other. You could also form two teams consisting of representatives from different departments, staff levels, or professional groups.

Setting up:

Form two teams of five people. Create question cards to use in the game, using questions from your training session. To fit the game's format, use questions that have only one or two correct answers.

How to play:

The host asks the two teams a question to start off the game. The first person to ring the buzzer (use bells, buzzers from board games, or horns) has the first opportunity to answer the question. If he or she answers correctly, then his or her team earns a point; if he or she answers incorrectly, the other team gets a chance to answer. The host continues asking questions until all the questions have been answered correctly. Have a suitable prize—such as a free pizza party—for the team that earns the most points.

Suggestion: Consider using this game as a "pop-quiz" to monitor awareness and understanding during the education or training session. It may also be an appropriate activity if learners are not following or understanding a concept.

CHAPTER 5

Events

CHAPTER 5

EVENTS

Events are another way to spice up learning for staff. By using extravagant booths and games, you'll get the complete attention of your staff. This will allow you to train them on the important care topics in a new and different way, keeping staff interested in the topic while fully engaging them in the learning process.

The following pages show you how to set up a carnival to make an exciting learning environment. Follow our lead or create your own carnival. Either way, remember to always have fun with your training!

Carnival

If you have the time and the energy to organize one, a carnival can be a fun, effective way to train staff on mandatory topics, such as infection control or Resident's Rights. It will give staff members the opportunity to learn about these topics in a new and exciting way and to interact with different departments.

Find out how large an area you can use to run the carnival—it will help you to determine how many booths you can have. You could use your auditorium, cafeteria, a few adjoining rooms, or an outdoor tent (depending on the weather). Plan to run your carnival from early in the morning until late at night—perhaps from 7 a.m. until 11 p.m.—to best ensure that all staff members have a chance to attend.

Select a theme for the carnival (e.g., baseball theme—see Figure 5.1, beach party, casino night, or Fourth of July) and have corresponding prizes, snacks, music, and decorations. A great way to utilize our game ideas is to hold a TV game show carnival. Use the talents of your staff members to help you organize the event and choose your topics. Consider using learners who did particularly well in training to help educate.

FIGURE 5.1 | **SAMPLE CARNIVAL BOOTHS AND IDEAS FOR A DAY AT THE BALLPARK**

To set up a carnival with a baseball theme do the following:

- Decorate your booths with posters in the shape of baseballs, baseball hats, pennants, and bats. Write educational information on the posters.

- Serve hot dogs, popcorn, peanuts, and boxes of Cracker Jack for snacks.

- Offer tickets to ball games, baseball hats with your organization's logo, or baseball cards as prizes.

Your carnival booths and games should have a baseball-related theme as well. Consider using the following two booths (see Figures 5.2 and 5.3) in your own organization's carnival.

Make sure that each booth focuses on a particular message and is not diluted with too much trivia. Each booth should include a game or other activity (following your carnival's theme) that quizzes staff members on its topic. The attendants of each booth could hang informational posters or have educational flyers available to help staff remember policies or important information. See Figures 5.2 and 5.3 for some sample carnival booths and ideas.

A week or two before your carnival, distribute information packets to staff describing the carnival events. Include material on the different booths and games and maybe a questionnaire to help staff prepare. Remind them that they will be tested on the information at the carnival.

To keep track of attendance and to ensure staff preparedness, have staff members bring their completed questionnaires to the carnival as their entrance tickets. The attendants of each booth should stamp the back of a staff member's questionnaire when he or she visits and plays the game. If the staff member does well, he or she should receive an extra stamp.

Have theme prizes available for attendees to win. The type of prize should depend on the number of stamps an attendee has earned. You could also have a theme raffle, using the questionnaires as tickets.

FIGURE **5.2**

SAMPLE BOOTH ONE: BATTER UP!

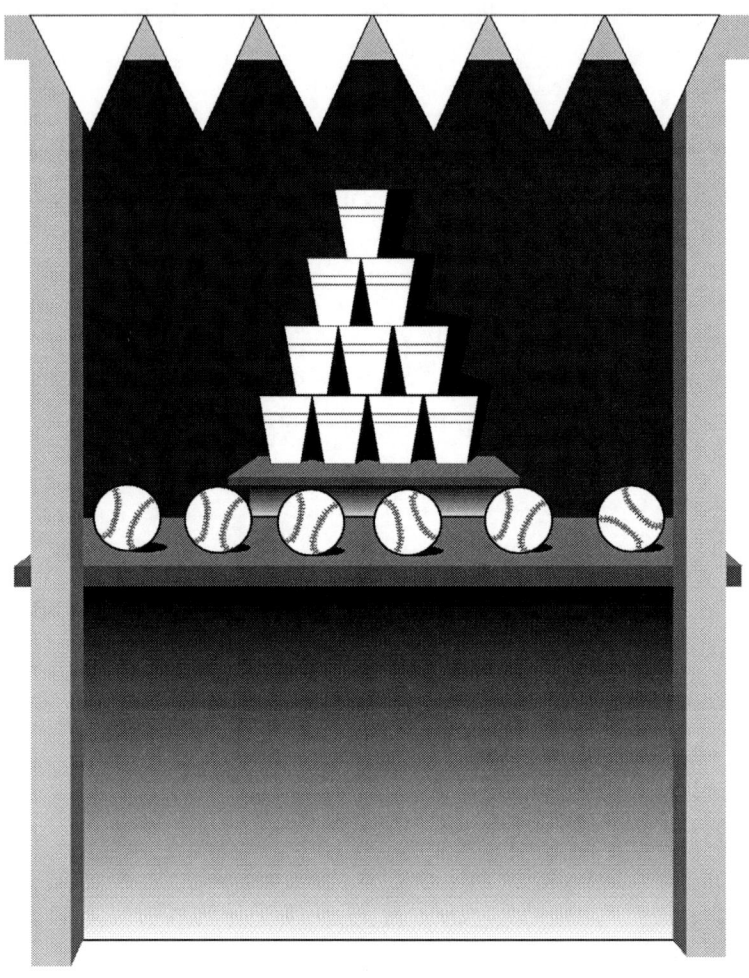

On a table against a wall or backdrop, make a stacked tower of plastic cups. On another table, line up six whiffle balls and number them from one to six. Place a question on your booth's topic under each ball and have participants answer all six questions. For each question the participant answers correctly, he or she gets to throw a ball to try to knock down the tower.

Stamp the back of the participant's quiz/entrance ticket to show that he or she visited the booth. Give an extra stamp for each question the participant answers correctly and/or each cup or bottle he or she knocks down. If the participant answers all six questions correctly, give him or her another stamp.

FIGURE **5.3** | **SAMPLE BOOTH TWO: THREE STRIKES AND YOU'RE OUT!**

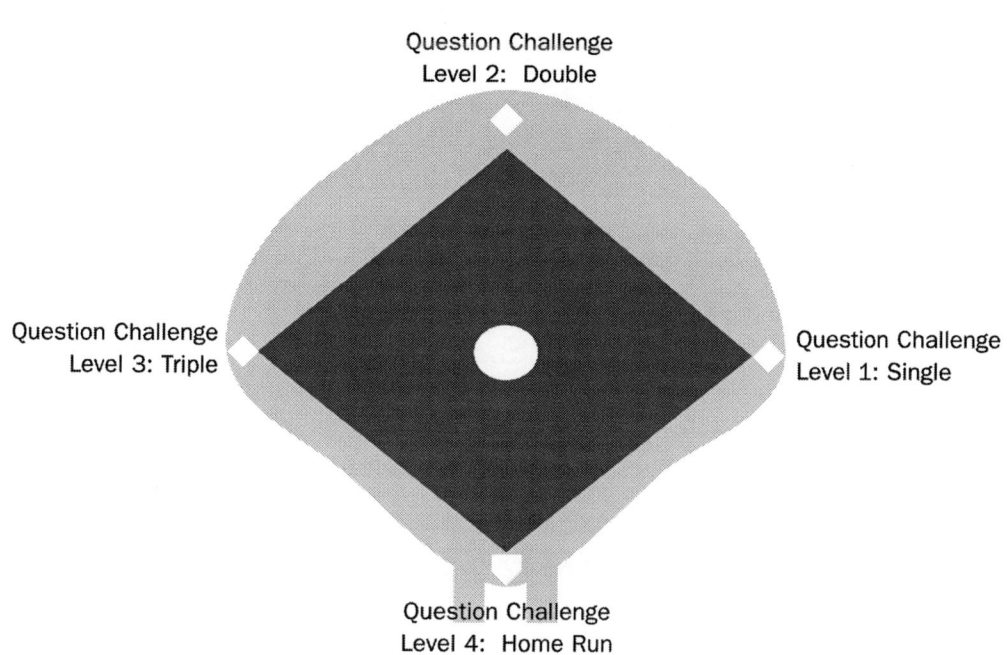

Question Challenge
Level 2: Double

Question Challenge
Level 3: Triple

Question Challenge
Level 1: Single

Question Challenge
Level 4: Home Run

For this booth's game, participants answer questions rated according to degree of difficulty. The degrees are measured in baseball terms—single, double, triple, home run, and grand slam. Participants get a point (or a stamp on the back of their quizzes) for answering a single question correctly, two points for correctly answering a double, and so forth. If a question has more than one correct answer, it is worth more points; the participant will receive a point for each answer that is correct. If a participant gets three strikes (i.e., answers three questions incorrectly), he or she is out of the game.

Participants can play this game individually or in teams—for example, have two departments, committees, or professional groups play against each other to encourage friendly competition. Set up a table with several chairs around it for participants to sit at and answer questions.

Have the teams play nine rounds, or innings, to determine a winner. Again, stamp the back of a participant's quiz/entrance ticket to show that he or she visited the booth. Consider giving winning teams extra stamps.

CHAPTER 6

Tools

CHAPTER 6

TOOLS

As a staff development coordinator, you will discover different ways to keep staff interested in training topics. Doing this requires you to use not only your imagination, but also any tool you can create to get staff to understand and retain the information you're teaching them in each inservice.

Flashcards are an example of a tool that is used to help staff memorize important information. The following pages contain examples of other tools you can use to help staff learn effectively.

Flashcards

Staff can use flashcards to review and test both their knowledge of each inservice topic and the policies and procedures that may accompany the lesson. Flashcards are easy to create, using 3 x 5 index cards or pieces of construction paper: Simply write a question on one side of a card and the answer on the other. You might want to separate cards according to focus area or staff level. You could also color-code them by category.

Have your learners use the flashcards to prepare for an education and training session. You could have learners create their own cards for those areas that continually give them trouble. You might also want to consider using the same flashcards for study purposes and for some of the games (such as Knowledge Bowl) to save time and effort.

Fun fact calendar

A calendar is a fun way to provide staff with important tips and information and is probably something that they will glance at daily. For each day on your calendar, include a fun fact, hint, tip, or question (with the answer) to help staff members remember important care and procedural facts. Make your calendar colorful and fun so staff members will enjoy reading each day's tip and look forward to the next. There are several calendar formats from which to choose:

- Using a standard month-per-page calendar, write a question or tip in each day's box. You can also create your own calendar with a large piece of colored posterboard.

- Another good format to use is the tear-away calendar. Create a page for each day out of construction paper or posterboard and write a question or tip on it.

- Create a calendar that looks like an Advent calendar: each day its own little door that opens to reveal a fact or tip. To make this calendar, use two pieces of posterboard, writing the facts or tips for each day on one piece and cutting out doors to match on the other. Creating this calendar requires a lot of imagination and a little skill with arts and crafts.

- If you don't have a lot of time to create a calendar, simply ask department managers to write each day's hint, tip, fact, or question on a chalkboard or dry-erase board with colorful chalk or markers.

Cheat sheets

Help your staff members "cheat"! For each inservice topic, create cheat sheets that include basic reminders, key policies and procedures, and need-to-know facts and tips. You could include a list, such as "The Top 10 Questions Every Caregiver Needs to Know," and you might also want to leave space for staff members to write notes and reminders. Your cheat sheet can be as simple as a 3 x 5 card or as complex as a tabbed booklet.

CHAPTER 7

Planning your inservice program

CHAPTER 7

PLANNING YOUR INSERVICE PROGRAM

Planning

Your facility's inservice training program must educate staff on the care and procedural topics they need to know in order to do their jobs well and offer residents quality care. Remember the following tips when planning your staff's yearly inservice program:

- **Stay organized.** As a staff development coordinator, you are responsible for the education and training of many people. This training must be documented so you will need to be organized while planning your inservices and while documenting this training for each staff member.

- **Design an inservice calendar.** Make up your inservice calendar for the year (Figure 7.1). First fill in the mandatory inservices, and then any other inservice in order of importance or urgency. Remember to take into consideration staff's suggestions for inservices and plan inservices around their needs.

- **Be prepared.** Make sure that you have enough of any handouts, prizes, or quizzes you provide for everyone in the inservice.

- **Stay on top of facility policies and procedures.** Keep your eyes and ears out for policy or procedure changes within your facility—you are responsible for educating or training staff on them.

- **Specify which staff should attend.** Know your audience's abilities when it comes to learning, and teach to their level. Confusing CNAs with procedures they will not need to perform or with language they don't understand will only frustrate them and make them not want to show up to the next inservice. Instead, teach separate inservices to separate groups when necessary. Also, keep staff's needs in mind when asking them to come to an inservice. If you know that a certain CNA has been having trouble with the topic you plan to train on, invite him or her to join the session.

- **Decide how you will handle documentation.** You are required to document staff's inservice training, so you will need to decide the best way to do so.

- **Keep tabs on staff's certification and recertification needs.** CNAs are required by each state to complete a certain number of training hours in order to remain certified. Find out the number for your state and keep track of each staff member's training. Doing so will allow you to remind them how their continuing education hours are coming along and whether or not they are in jeopardy of losing their certification, which would mean they can no longer legally practice as a caregiver.

- **Work within your means.** Keep your budget, time, and resources for training in mind whenever planning an inservice.

- **Keep management in the loop.** Regularly inform management (and others who may be interested) of the status of your facility's staff education and training efforts.

Thorough planning will help you execute strong, informative inservices from which staff will learn important lessons. Try to anticipate staff's questions and concerns before beginning the session. When considering topics for your inservices, ask yourself the following five questions:

1. Who is this topic going to be important to?
2. What problem will the inservice address?
3. Where will staff use this information?
4. When do staff need to know this information by?
5. Why do staff need this training?

FIGURE 7.1 | **SAMPLE INSERVICE CALENDAR**

Month	CNA education topics	Nursing education topics	Both	Competencies	Other
January	• Ethics and professionalism • Psychotropic meds	OSHA forms	Side-rail entrapment prevention	IVs	
February	• Safe lifts, transfers, and mobility assists • UTIs	Failure modes and effect analysis (FMEA)	Disaster drill	Combative residents	
March	• Pain management • Vision impairment	Digital radiology	Laundry issues	CPR	
April	• HIPAA: Privacy, confidentiality, and security • Review of the respiratory system	Chemicals and labeling	Mechanical-lifts training	Oxygen	
May	• Skin problems and care • Elder abuse	Education assessment	Door alarm		
June	• Infection control • Survey preparation	Medication documentation	Communication skills		
July	• Falls prevention • Vital signs	ICD-9 coding		Tracheostomy care	
August	• Resident's Rights, restraints, and confidentiality • Vision impairment	(1) CP update	Elopement system		
September	• Bloodborne pathogens • Alzheimer's disease	(2) CP update		CLIA and pain assessment (nurses)	
October	• End-of-life care • Depression and anxiety	BiPAP	Fire and safety		
November	• Effects of aging • Influenza (flu)	MDS updates		Competencies (CNAs)	
December	• Seizure disorders • Foot health	Needle safety	Chemical and biological terrorism	Competencies (licensed staff)	

 Also appears on your CD-ROM.

CHAPTER 8

Inservice training

CHAPTER 8

INSERVICE TRAINING

Documenting training

In addition to providing continuous education and training for your CNAs, you are also required to document it.

Any time policies and procedures change, staff must be promptly trained on the change. When new staff members are hired and require orientation, they must be trained as well. Because these trainings are required, you must document them to prove that they've occurred.

In fact, it is important to document which staff members have been educated and trained on every topic. Doing so not only helps you plan your educational efforts but also provides important evidence should your organization need to show that it has properly educated and trained its staff members.

Ask all learners to complete a quiz following each inservice to document their basic understanding of the training. Learner quizzes are located on the CD-ROM, while the answer keys can be found at the beginning of each inservice in this manual.

Reward your inservice participants with certificates that document their completion of your organization's education and training program. Awarding such certificates:

- Shows staff members that you appreciate the time they've taken to learn about different care topics
- Demonstrates the importance of each topic
- Produces another document that serves as evidence that your organization educates its caregivers

Depending on how your organization prefers to document education and training, you may keep documentation in a number of different ways:

- Keep either a paper or an electronic log of education and training completed and documents provided (see Figure 8.1). Binders and filing cabinets with folders for each staff member are good, organized ways to store documentation.

- Keep paper copies of the completed learner quizzes, and add the exam scores to your education and training log. You may need to refer to them if questioned by surveyors or others regarding staff's training.

- Keep copies of learner evaluations. Sample learner evaluations are provided in Chapter 10 of this manual.

At a minimum, you should track:

- Learner name
- Department
- Inservice topic
- Date of the inservice

Tracking CNAs' training hours

Keep track of the number of training hours each CNA has completed. Doing so is important because the state determines the amount of hours of training CNAs must have, and if they fail to meet the annual training requirements, they will lose their certification and no longer be able to legally work as caregivers. By helping CNAs keep track of these important training hours, you ensure that none lose or even risk losing their certification.

This chapter includes a sample of a training reminder note (see Figure 8.1), which informs caregivers of how many training hours they have, how many they must receive to remain certified, and the date by which they must complete their training. Hand reminders to staff while inviting them to join you at the next inservice. Otherwise, find another way to get the reminder note to them so they do not risk losing their certification. (Training reminder notes are customizable and printable, and are located on your CD-ROM).

Remember, do not reprimand CNAs for needing more training hours. Instead, help them reach this goal by being available to them as an educator and professional guide. Remind them that they are important to their residents and that you want them to stay in your facility—or "family."

FIGURE 8.1

SAMPLE TRAINING REMINDER NOTE

WE WANT YOU IN OUR FAMILY!

Name:

Date:

Completed training hours: _____

Amount of training hours still needed: _____

Date training hours must be completed by: _____

Remember, if you don't meet the state requirements for certification, you can no longer legally practice as a CNA in this state. Please don't let that happen—we want you in our family!

Please join us for the next inservice! Check out the details:

_____

Also appears on your CD-ROM.

CHAPTER 9

Follow-up training

CHAPTER 9

FOLLOW-UP TRAINING

In order to ensure that training has been successful, you need to assess the success of the education and training and assess how the learners felt about the training.

Assessing training success

To assess the success of the education and training, you need to ask two questions:

- Were the stated learning objectives accomplished?
- Has the new knowledge been successfully applied to the job?

Basically, these two questions assess the same thing: whether the learners successfully learned and retained the information from the training session. The difference between them is that one assesses success in the short term (i.e., during and immediately following the training) and the other assesses success in the long term (i.e., defined as appropriately using the training in the day-to-day activities).

Short-term success

To assess short-term success, monitor awareness and understanding as you work through the education and training session. Quizzes, games, and interaction such as question-and-answer sessions are good ways to do so. Include a quiz at the end of the education and training to make sure that the learners accomplished the training goals.

Long-term success

You can assess the long-term success either by directly following up with the learners or by querying learners' managers.

If you plan to follow up with the learners, consider sending out a brief questionnaire that includes sample situations and questions to assess retention and knowledge application. Make sure that staff members know that their answers will not have negative consequences—to that end, you might consider making the questionnaire anonymous. The answers—with or without knowing whose they are—will let you identify whether the appropriate number of people have adequately retained the training. This plan will require buy-in from managers because they will need to approve staff member time spent on this task.

Another way to assess long-term success is to ask a learner's manager a few questions to see whether the learner is applying the education and training. Or you might provide a list of the learner's activities for the manager to assess.

Tell the managers and learners that you are available to answer any questions. Manager buy-in and knowledge of the education and training is essential. Consider providing additional resources for managers to use in assisting their work force as they apply the training.

Assessing how the learners felt about the training

An education and training program needs to be dynamic, evolving as the information and the learners' needs change. Additionally, as you educate and train, you will find that some methods work and some methods don't. Find ways to refine your program so that it better achieves your learning objectives. Getting learner feedback is one of the best methods of discovering how you can make your education and training program as relevant and learner-oriented as possible, as well as how to focus it on accomplishing your training goals.

Consider using forms that ask the learners to both rate the education and training and rate you as the trainer. You can use the forms separately or you may combine them. Samples of these forms are included in this manual (see Chapter 10).

Providing feedback to the learners

Just as your best source of feedback is your learners, one of the best ways for your learners to be sure that they have achieved all of their education and training goals is for you to provide useful and effective feedback to them. You can accomplish this task indirectly by using learning-retention training techniques. Do this by surprising staff members with a question or two regarding a recent inservice. Or, take five minutes before your next inservice to review important points from the previous inservice. Use flashcards to make the quick review session more interactive.

CHAPTER 10

Learner evaluations

CHAPTER 10

| LEARNER EVALUATIONS |

As mentioned earlier, obtaining learner feedback is vital for understanding whether the education and training you're giving staff is informative and useful. Finding out how learners feel about your inservices will allow you to mold the sessions around their learning abilities, making better use of your training efforts. Asking learners about the education and training you're providing, and the training techniques you're implementing, will only strengthen you as a staff development coordinator.

They love the inservice, they love it not

Consider using forms that ask the learners to rate both the education and training and you as the trainer. You can use the forms separately or you may combine them.

Continuously apply the information you obtain through learner evaluations, even if it means adjusting duplicate sessions. You must lead to reach everyone in your staff. Don't be afraid to improve your presentation and selection of tools as you go along—use learner evaluations to help in crafting improvements. Also realize that some learner reactions may be important enough to impact your whole education and training plan. For instance, if learners feel they are missing the message or becoming confused because too much information is covered, you may want to consider adding follow-up training mechanisms to reinforce key points. To prepare for this possibility, conduct a trial education and training session early in your schedule with a pilot group of learners to gather feedback that can help you craft the most effective program possible before rollout.

Sample form A: Rate the trainer

Note: Have staff complete this form at the conclusion of the inservice. Feel free to alter the questions so that they reflect your training program. These forms are included on the CD-ROM in the "Instructor aids" folder. Based on your knowledge of both your organization and your learners, you can ask for personal details, such as name and job, or make the form anonymous. Figure 10.1 gives a sample of an anonymous form.

Recommendation: Consider handing out this form at the beginning of the inservice and asking learners to look over the questions. Doing so will give them an idea of what to observe during training.

FIGURE 10.1 — SAMPLE FORM A: RATE THE TRAINER

Title of inservice: Trainer:
Date of inservice: Location of inservice
Name of trainer: or event:

Your feedback is very important. Please let us know what you thought of the inservice so that we may continue to develop training that best suits your needs. Thank you for your opinions.

Please circle a number for the questions below:

Statement	Never		Sometimes		Always
Demonstrated strong knowledge about the subject matter	1	2	3	4	5
Appeared well-prepared to instruct	1	2	3	4	5
Used visual materials, handouts, and activities effectively	1	2	3	4	5
Gave clear, concise explanations	1	2	3	4	5
Solicited questions and had the answers	1	2	3	4	5
Demonstrated an interest in sharing information and knowledge	1	2	3	4	5
Demonstrated the ability to communicate well with learners	1	2	3	4	5
Displayed patience	1	2	3	4	5
Effectively explained each topic	1	2	3	4	5
Appropriately allocated time for each topic	1	2	3	4	5
Allowed for different learning styles and speeds	1	2	3	4	5
Geared material appropriately for learner needs	1	2	3	4	5

What improvements could the trainer make to his/her style or to the inservice session?

Consider the trainer's skills. Which is/are the strongest? Which is/are the weakest?

Your feedback is valuable. Please feel free to provide further comments below:

 Also appears on your CD-ROM.

Sample form B: Rate the training

Note: Have staff complete this form at the conclusion of the inservice. Based on your knowledge of both your organization and your learners, you can ask for personal details, such as name and job, or make the form anonymous. Figure 10.2 gives a sample of an anonymous form.

Recommendation: Consider handing out this form at the beginning of the inservice and asking staff to look over the questions. Doing so will give them an idea of what to observe during training.

FIGURE 10.2 | SAMPLE FORM B: RATE THE TRAINING

Title of inservice:

Date of inservice:

Name of trainer:

Trainer:

Location of inservice

or event:

Your feedback is very important. Please let us know what you thought of the inservice so that we may continue to develop training that best suits your needs. Thank you for your opinions.

Please circle a number for the questions below:

Statement	Not at all		A little		Completely
This inservice session met my training goals	1	2	3	4	5
This inservice session met the overall course goals	1	2	3	4	5
This inservice session provided me with the information I need to do my job	1	2	3	4	5
I understood why I needed this training	1	2	3	4	5
I understood the material presented	1	2	3	4	5

How would you rate the organization of this event?

Excellent   Good   Okay   Poor   Very poor

How would you rate your level of interest in the material?

Excellent   Good   Okay   Poor   Very poor

How would you rate your level of interest during the presentation?

Excellent   Good   Okay   Poor   Very poor

How would you rate the pace of the event?

Excellent   Good   Okay   Poor   Very poor

If any of your personal training goals or overall course goals were not met, please specify those that were not met:

If you particularly liked or did not like some of the elements or activities during the inservice, please specify which they were:

What were the main benefits of the inservice, and what did you learn that was most valuable?

Indicate how your performance in your job might improve as a result of attending this inservice:

Your constructive feedback is very helpful. Please feel free to provide any further comments below:

 Also appears on your CD-ROM.

CHAPTER 11

Lesson plans

LESSON PLANS

1. Activities and exercise

2. Caring for residents with dementia

3. Depression and anxiety

4. Diabetes

5. Incontinence

6. Malnutrition and dehydration

7. Elopement and wandering

8. Mental illness

9. Communication guidelines

10. Coping with death

Activities and exercise

Overview

This lesson is designed to help workers who care for adults of all ages in a variety of settings.

Program time
Approximately 45 minutes

Learning objectives
After completing this lesson, participants will be able to do the following:

- Explain the benefits of being socially, mentally, and physically active throughout life
- Promote activity and exercise and encourage clients to participate
- Describe the risks of different types of activities and the precautions necessary for safe activity
- List exercise recommendations for intensity, duration, and frequency
- Guide adults in safely performing several different types of activities and exercises

Preparation

1. Familiarize yourself with the information by reviewing the lesson prior to teaching it.

2. Print and pass out appropriate handout(s) when instructed.

3. Print out a quiz and certificate for each learner from the CD-ROM.

Method

1. Deliver a mini-lecture covering the material in the workbook on pages 1–4. To make teaching easier, use the instruction icons as cues for leading the session. Be sure to insert your facility's policies and procedures whenever appropriate.

2. Encourage participant discussion when appropriate, and ask for additional ideas to help handle difficult behavior from residents with Alzheimer's disease.

3. Hand out the quiz and allow adequate time for each participant to finish.

4. Give certificates of completion to those who correctly answered at least seven of the questions.

Answer key

1. A	4. D	7. C	10. True
2. C	5. D	8. False	
3. B	6. C	9. False	

Activities and exercise

Activities and exercise are critical to the well-being of your residents. People who regularly interact socially with others tend to be healthier, both physically and mentally, than those who become socially isolated. Recreational activities improve motor skills, social skills, thinking ability, behavior, and communication ability. Artistic activities such as arts and crafts help people relax, keep an alert mind, improve fine motor skills, and improve memory. All types of activities prevent boredom and loneliness, and promote choice and independence.

 Activities and you

To personalize this lesson and help staff members better understand the importance of activities, have each person share with the group activities he or she is involved in personally and explain why they are important to him or her.

Physical activity

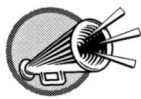 *Read through the following items related to the importance of physical activity.*

Physical activity is an important part of our resident's care. It can:

- Reduce risk of heart disease.

- Help with weight control.

- Improve blood circulation.

- Decrease the risk of falls.

- Relieve symptoms of anxiety and depression.

- Help prevent and control chronic diseases such as high blood pressure, diabetes, and osteoporosis. It also lowers cholesterol.

- Improve gross motor skills and help residents maintain independence in self-care.

- Strengthen heart and lungs.

- Improve the mobility, balance, and coordination.

- Increase flexibility of joints and muscles.

- Improves self-esteem and quality of life.

- Improve strength and endurance.

- Prevent muscle atrophy and contractures.

- Keep people functional. Physical activity helps them be able to get up out of chairs, walk, eat, and bathe without assistance for as long as possible.

These benefits are even <u>more</u> important for older and disabled people. Even very weak and frail people can improve their strength, endurance, and ability to do things by exercising regularly.

 *Pass out the "Recommendations for Regular Physical Exercise" handout to participants.*

Aged and disabled people often don't move much for long periods of time. When their muscles are not exercised, they can waste away, or atrophy. When this happens, the muscles become small and weak. The muscles can also tighten up into deformities called contractures. When this happens, the muscles stop working. In addition, lack of exercise weakens the body and body systems. These problems lead to dependence on others, inability to do self-care, and poorer quality of life.

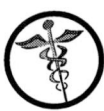 *Any kind of exercise or activity is better than doing nothing at all.*

Recommendations for Regular Physical Exercise

Type of Exercise	Benefits	How	How Much (Intensity)	How Long (Duration)	How Often (Frequency)
Aerobic Exercise	Strengthens heart and lungs, increases stamina and endurance, helps with weight control, and improves circulation.	Aerobic exercises include walking, dancing, and calisthenics. Low impact calisthenics, with no jumping, are safest. An easy exercise for an older person is marching in place.	Aerobic exercise is based on increasing oxygen intake to stimulate heart and lung activity. For an exercise to be aerobic it must increase heart rate and breathing above a person's normal rates (but not too high).	Thirty minutes to one hour. This time can be broken up into shorter ten-minute sessions with many of the same benefits of a longer session. Three ten-minute sessions spaced out over a day might be the best routine for an older person.	At least three times a week.
Muscle Building and Toning (Anaerobic Exercise)	Increases strength, improves appearance, increases mobility, improves ability to do self-care, improves coordination and balance, and decreases the risk of falls.	Lift light weights (start with one-pound weights and increase slowly). Do muscle-toning calisthenics such as squats and leg raises. Gardening is a fun muscle-building activity	Lift the weights or do the muscle-toning calisthenics in sets of eight repetitions, and repeat each set twice. Adjust the size of the weight to be able to perform all the repetitions without harm. It may be necessary to start with just two or three repetitions.	Work up to twenty to thirty minutes. Start with just a few lifts or calisthenics, and increase slowly over time.	Twice a week, or every other day. Always allow at least 48 hours between muscle-building sessions.
Stretching and Range of Motion (ROM)	Increases flexibility, prevents injury, and helps the joints and muscles keep or recover functioning.	ROM gently moves the joints through all types of movement. Stretching pulls gently on the muscles.	ROM and stretching can be active, done by the client, or passive, done by a caregiver. Active-assisted is done partly by the client, with assistance. Clients should do as much of the work as they can.	Five minutes is enough for a post-exercise stretch. If stretching or range of motion is the only exercise being performed, work for fifteen to twenty minutes (or longer) if possible.	Every day, or at least five times a week.

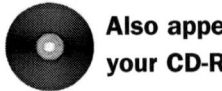 **Also appears on your CD-ROM.**

Promoting exercise and activities

You are responsible for helping the people you take care of be as active, independent, and healthy as possible. Become a "cheerleader" for activity and exercise. Know how important it is to stay active, and try to motivate people to engage in some kind of activity or exercise every day.

People have the right to choose their activities. Never force anyone to do something they don't want to do—but you can explain how important activity is.

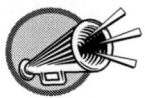

Ask staff how they encourage residents to participate in activities, and then share with them the following suggestions.

You can encourage residents to participate in activities and exercise in the following ways:

- Tell them about some of the many emotional and mental benefits of socialization and activity.

- Emphasize that they can choose the activities they like and that they may stop performing an activity or quit participating in a social event whenever they wish.

- Find out what a resident likes to do. What hobbies does he or she enjoy? What kind of music? What kind of art? Encourage continued involvement in these things as much as possible. If you need additional materials for these activities, work with your supervisor to obtain them.

- If a resident has given up a hobby he or she enjoyed due to poor vision or motor skills, see if there are adaptive devices that can help. A magnifying glass that attaches to a book or needlework frame can enable someone to see well enough to read or stitch.

- Sometimes a formerly loved hobby can be modified so an elderly or disabled person can still do it. If someone used to like to sew but can't handle the tiny needle and thread now, perhaps they could manage the large tapestry needles and thick yarns used in plastic canvas needlework. Be creative!

- Bring residents with similar interests together. People who like plants would enjoy looking at each other's flowers or greenery and sharing knowledge, stories, and ideas about growing things.

• Help provide the things people need to do an activity they have chosen. If they want to do a jigsaw puzzle, find a way to get them some puzzles they can do.

Safety precautions

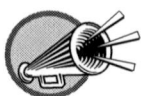 *Explain to staff the importance of monitoring residents during activities. Share with them your facility's policies and procedures for reporting accidents.*

When you are working with someone who has a physical or mental disability, the risk of injury or harm during an activity increases. Here are some things to watch for and some precautions to observe:

 ! Safety tip

No one with dementia, suicidal tendencies, cognitive impairment, or a history of violent behavior should use a sharp or pointed object unless you are able to provide constant supervision.

Arts and crafts

The tools used in a craft project can be dangerous if used improperly. Scissors, knives, sewing needles, knitting needles, and other sharp or pointed objects can cause cuts, punctures, and eye injuries.

Cooking projects

Stoves and ovens create a risk for burns. Microwave ovens carry the risk of steam burns. Hot foods and liquids can cause serious burns if mishandled or spilled. Small household appliances, such as mixers, can be a source of electric shock or injuries. Knives, scissors, and other cooking utensils can cause cuts and punctures.

Safety tip

Forgetfulness, poor motor skills, and muscle weakness put a person at risk of forgetting about or mishandling a hot food, object, or appliance, so cooking must be closely supervised for people that are cognitively impaired, frail, or uncoordinated in their movements. Observe safety rules for sharp objects.

Safety tip

Watch for signs of anxiety, anger, hostility, or frustration during a game or mental activity. If someone becomes upset, intervene with assistance or redirect the person to another activity. Try to help the individual quietly and avoid calling attention to the problem if possible. Foster a sense of control by offering a variety of activities and asking the person to choose one.

Games and mental activities

If a mental activity or game is too difficult for someone, they may become frustrated or angry. Sometimes a person will act out this anger or frustration with unpleasant or inappropriate behavior or speech. Self-esteem and confidence might be reduced, and people may become anxious or depressed as a result.

Safety tip

Explain what is going to happen before beginning a social activity or outing. Be sure that any rules or restrictions are applied fairly and evenly to all the people involved in the activity.

If you observe a conflict, stop the activity and separate the individuals involved. Gently redirect them. Focus on the pleasant aspects of the activity and shift attention away from the conflict.

Social activities

Any interaction between people carries the risk of disagreements, jealousy, excessive competitiveness, unfair actions, and other conflict that can create a negative atmosphere and make the activity unpleasant for others.

QUIZ

Activities and exercise

Name: _____

Date: _____ Score: _____

Directions: Circle the correct answer to the questions below.

1. **Some benefits of social activities include:**
   a. Reduced boredom, loneliness, and depression
   b. Increased balance and coordination
   c. Reduced risk of heart disease
   d. Decreased risk of falls

2. **Some benefits of physical exercise include:**
   a. Improved communication ability
   b. Less likelihood of dementia
   c. Increased strength and flexibility
   d. Improved thinking ability

3. **If a resident doesn't want to do an activity you suggest, you should:**
   a. Insist that the resident participate and tell him it's for his own good.
   b. Respect the resident's right to refuse, and offer another activity he might enjoy more.
   c. Tell your supervisor that the resident is uncooperative.
   d. Tell the resident you are upset with her for refusing.

4. **Active-assisted range of motion means:**
   a. Range of motion exercises performed completely by the resident
   b. Range of motion exercises performed completely by the caregiver
   c. Range of motion exercises performed by a therapist or nurse
   d. Range of motion exercises performed partly by the resident, with assistance from a caregiver

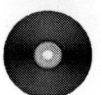 **Also appears on your CD-ROM.**

Activities and exercise (cont.)

QUIZ

5. **When muscles are not used:**
    a. They can waste away or atrophy, becoming small and weak
    b. They can tighten up into contractures and stop working
    c. Neither a nor b
    d. Both a and b

6. **You can encourage a resident to participate in activities by**
    a. Forcing him or her to join in an activity
    b. Tell he or she will be punished if he or she doesn't participate
    c. Emphasize that he or she can choose the activities he or she likes and that he or she may stop performing an activity or quit participating in a social event whenever he or she wishes.
    d. Bring him or her to whichever activity is most convenient for your schedule

7. **If a resident tells you she would enjoy doing a hobby she likes if she had the supplies, what should you do?**
    a. Nothing. It's not your place to provide hobby supplies.
    b. Tell the resident that the hobby would be too difficult for her now.
    c. Offer to help the resident obtain the supplies, or inform the family or your supervisor.
    d. Purchase the supplies yourself and give them to the resident.

8. **Since people can become frustrated when working a puzzle or other mental activity, it is best to avoid activities that require the resident to think.**
    True or False

9. **If a resident can't exercise for at least thirty minutes a day, he might as well not bother to do it at all, since it won't do any good to exercise for shorter periods of time.**
    True or False

10. **If a resident doesn't want to participate in an activity, you cannot force him or her to, but you can explain how important the activity.**
    True or False

CERTIFICATE OF COMPLETION

This is to certify that

_____

has read and successfully passed the final exam of

Activities and exercise

_____

Supervisor name

Caring for residents with dementia

Overview

This lesson teaches useful ways to work with residents who suffer from dementia.

Program time

Approximately 45 minutes

Learning objectives

After completing this lesson, participants will be able to do the following:

- Know the definition and symptoms of dementia

- Know some good ways to respond to difficult behavior

- Know the importance of trying to understand what a resident with dementia is thinking and feeling

- Understand the difficulties faced by someone with dementia

Preparation

1. Familiarize yourself with the information by reviewing the lesson prior to teaching it.

2. Print and pass out appropriate handout(s) when instructed.

3. Print out a quiz and certificate for each learner from the CD-ROM.

Method

1. Deliver a mini-lecture covering the material in the workbook on pages 5–8. To make teaching easier, use the instruction icons as cues for leading the session. Be sure to insert your facility's policies and procedures whenever appropriate.

2. Ask a learner to read the definition and causes of dementia from the learning guide. See if the learners have any questions about this information.

3. Briefly review the "Important things to remember about dementia" on the learning guide. Mention that it might seem time-consuming to try to figure out what a resident with dementia is thinking or feeling, but residents have the right to expect this from their care-givers. In addition, spending the time to do this will often save time and difficulty later.

Emphasize that there is not one right way to help, but that each individual person has special needs and special ways of relating that must be understood.

4. Ask three different learners to present one of the case studies to the group. Allow for discussion.

5. Play the bingo game by calling out the test questions and letting the learners find the answers on their game cards.

6. Hand out the quiz and allow adequate time for each participant to finish.

7. Give certificates of completion to those who correctly answered at least seven of the questions.

Answer key

1. H	5. E	9. F
2. I	6. C	10. K
3. A	7. G	11. L
4. M	8. B	12. D

Understanding dementia

Dementia is a mental disorder involving a general loss of intellectual abilities and changes in the personality. Many different things cause dementia. The most common, in order of occurrence, are:

1. Alzheimer's disease

2. Strokes and other blood vessel diseases

3. Parkinson's and other nervous system diseases

4. Miscellaneous causes such as alcoholism, malnutrition, head injuries, drug reactions, thyroid disease, brain tumors, and infections

The results of dementia

Dementia can have the following effects on residents:

1. **Memory loss**

    • Affects recent memories the most

    • Makes it difficult to learn anything new or to follow instructions

2. **Language loss (the meaning of words)**

    • Makes it difficult to recognize words and understand complex sentences

    • Makes if difficult to express ideas

3. **Attention loss**

    • Unable to start or stop a task

    • Easily distracted

4. **Judgment loss**

    • Cannot accurately assess circumstances

    • Unable to see consequences of actions

5. Loss of perception or senses

- Unable to recognize things or people

- Misinterpret what they see, hear, or feel

6. Loss of muscle organization

- Unable to perform multiple-step tasks

- Require prompts or cues for routine tasks

 ## Dementia misconceptions

To personalize this lesson, ask staff members to share some misconceptions people unfamiliar with the disorder have abut dementia.

 ## Important things to remember about dementia

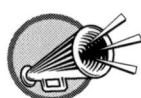 *Read through the following tips about dealing with residents with dementia. Stress the importance of being compassionate and understanding.*

- Adult dementia sufferers deserve the respect and status they have earned. They often do not know their abilities have changed, and do not understand why people treat them differently. They must be given as many opportunities as possible to make decisions and retain control over their lives.

- With the right environment and support, a resident's ability to function can be strengthened and improved. If those supports are removed, the resident's function will decline.

- The deficiencies caused by dementia affect all areas of a person's life. Although the disability is invisible, it affects the resident's ability to do even the smallest activities.

- The way a person with dementia behaves is not just the result of impaired brain functions. Behavior is often caused by efforts to meet needs while compensating for lost abilities.

- We can help people with dementia by trying to understand what they feel and think.

 *Pass out and review the "Communication tips" handout.*

Communication tips

✔ Be open, friendly, and gentle at all times.

✔ Always address the person by name to get his attention at the beginning of an interaction.

✔ Give your full attention to the conversation or task. This helps the resident stay focused.

✔ Briefly introduce yourself and offer some cues when you approach, stating your name and relationship and the purpose of your visit.

✔ Speak slowly, but do not speak down.

✔ Use gentle touching or hand holding, but get permission first.

✔ Avoid arguing and attempts to reason with a person who is upset. Acknowledge his feelings and calmly distract him with something calming, pleasant, and friendly.

 Also appears on your CD-ROM.

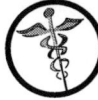 ## Ways to help a resident perform a task

Residents with dementia may have difficulty performing day-to-day tasks. However, there are certain things we can do to help them.

1. Explain each step in simple language, one thing at a time.

2. Demonstrate each step, doing the task while he or she watches.

3. Move the person through the steps of the task, placing arms and legs in the right positions.

4. If distracted, begin again at the beginning.

Remember to be patient and unhurried!

Case studies

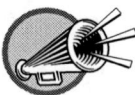

Have a learner read each of the case studies aloud to the rest of the group. After each is read, encourage learners to discuss "what caregivers assume" and "what is really happening." After learners have shared their opinions, review the answers provided in the manual.

Case study 1

Mrs. Allen is usually cooperative and pleasant. One day you find her wandering through a hallway far from her room, opening room doors and trying to get out an exit door. When you try to steer her back to her room, she becomes resistant, standing still and loudly shouting that she won't go with you. When you take her hand to guide her along, she swings at you with her other hand.

What caregivers may assume: Mrs. Allen must be progressing in her disease and should now be classified as "aggressive." She may need additional medication or evaluation in a hospital.

What is really happening: Mrs. Allen is thirsty (changes in the brain often make people with dementia very thirsty). She knows something is wrong and that she needs something, but she doesn't understand the sensation she is feeling. She also doesn't know how to meet the need, or what she should do to find water. So she is wandering the halls, looking for some cue that will help her know what she needs to do. When you try to prevent this activity, she naturally becomes angry at your efforts to keep her from meeting an important need. She feels she is defending herself from someone who is trying to harm her.

Try this: Help Mrs. Allen figure out what she needs. Ask questions to determine why she is wandering around. Did she lose something? Is she hungry? Is she thirsty? Does she need company? Is she bored? Make the questions simple and direct, allowing for yes or no answers. If she cannot answer your questions, try bringing her a class of water or a piece of fruit. Check to see if she has soiled her clothing or needs to change into dry clothes. Once you have determined what Mrs. Allen needs and have met that need, she is more likely to return to her normal activities.

Case study 2

Mr. Blair is not normally incontinent. Recently, however, he has begun walking outside to relieve himself. Sometimes the workers find he has urinated in his wastebasket. Occasionally he wets himself. He has started to wander, and he often seems anxious and agitated.

What caregivers may assume: Mr. Blair has lost the ability to control his bladder and should be placed in adult incontinent briefs.

What is really happening: Mr. Blair cannot find the toilet. In this facility the white toilets blend in with the cream-colored tiles and walls, and his visual loss is causing him to be unable to see them. He spends much of the day looking for a place to urinate, but when he can't find one he relieves himself outside or in a wastebasket, most of which are brightly colored and easy to see.

Try this: Place a brightly colored toilet seat or toilet cover on Mr. Blair's commode to help him locate it. When you see Mr. Blair wandering anxiously in the halls or acting agitated, ask if you can help him find a bathroom and then guide him to one.

Case study 3

Miss Mead was a nurse for forty years. She is new to your facility, and she refuses to eat in the dining room but insists on having a tray brought to her room. She doesn't eat the food you bring, but places the dishes on her windowsills and cabinets "for the others." She is losing weight rapidly but refuses to eat.

What caregivers may assume: Miss Mead will have to be placed in a hospital and fed with a stomach tube because of her refusal to eat.

What is really happening: Miss Mead is concerned for the "others" that she sees in her room. She believes that her reflections in the mirrors and windows are actually people that need her to care for them. She will not eat until she feeds them first.

Try this: Ask questions to determine what Miss Mead is trying to do. Once you understand the situation, remove the mirrors from Miss Mead's room. Cover the windows with blinds or shades. You could provide two trays of food, one for Miss Mead and one for "the others."

Caring for residents with dementia

Name: _____

Date: _____   **Score:** _____

Matching Test. Find the answer that best matches each situation.
You will not use all the answers.

1. In the case study about Mr. Blair, the caregivers helped him by providing what? _____

2. Mr. Sims was a plant supervisor for most of his life. He is very unhappy in your facility, but his dementia makes it impossible for him to live alone. What intervention might help him adjust to living in the residence? _____

3. We can help people with dementia by doing what? _____

4. Many times a person with dementia behaves in a difficult fashion because he or she is trying to: _____

5. When a person with dementia can't remember how to get in to a car or get dressed, which of the six "Results of Dementia" is causing the problem? _____

6. You should do this when starting a conversation with a resident with dementia. _____

7. When a person can't think of a word, or the words come out wrong or in the wrong order, they are experiencing which of the six "Results of Dementia?" _____

8. This is one way to help a person with dementia perform a task. _____

9. It is important that persons with dementia be allowed to do this as much as possible. _____

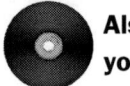 **Also appears on your CD-ROM.**

Caring for residents with dementia (cont.)

QUIZ

10. It is best to use these kinds of questions when dealing with residents with dementia. _____

11. Dementia is a condition that is characterized by: _____

12 We should try not to embarrass people with dementia, but instead treat them with: _____

A. Putting ourselves in their shoes, trying to understand what they feel and think
B. Tell the person how to do each step in simple language, one thing at a time
C. Address the person by name, and briefly introduce yourself and state the purpose of your visit
D. Respect
E. Loss of muscle organization
F. Make decisions and retain control over their lives
G. Language loss
H. Strong visual cues (contrasting colors on things the resident uses)
I. Ask him to give you regular reports on the activities in the facility, giving him a feeling of responsibility similar to the work he did in his career
J. Ask him to quit complaining and try to be happy
K. Direct, closed questions such as "Would you like to wear this red dress today?" instead of open-ended questions like "What would you like to wear today?"
L. Loss of intellectual abilities and personality changes
M. Cope with or compensate for lost abilities

CERTIFICATE OF COMPLETION

This is to certify that

_____

has read and successfully passed the final exam of

Caring for residents with dementia

_____

Supervisor name

Depression and anxiety

Overview

This lesson is designed to help workers recognize the signs and symptoms of depression.

Program time
Approximately 45 minutes

Learning objectives
After completing this lesson, participants will be able to do the following:

- Be able to define depression and anxiety and their causes

- Know the signs and symptoms of depression and anxiety

- Know some ways to prevent depression and anxiety

- Know how to care for people with depression or anxiety

- Know the warning signs of suicide and how to prevent it

Preparation

1. Familiarize yourself with the information by reviewing the lesson prior to teaching it.
2. Print and pass out appropriate handout(s) when instructed.
3. Print out a quiz and certificate for each learner from the CD-ROM.

Method

1. Deliver a mini-lecture covering the material in the workbook on pages 9–14. To make teaching easier, use the instruction icons as cues for leading the session. Be sure to insert your facility's policies and procedures whenever appropriate.
2. Encourage participant discussion when appropriate.
3. Hand out the quiz and allow adequate time for each participant to finish.
4. Give certificates of completion to those who correctly answered at least seven of the questions.

Answer key

1. D	4. A	7. Both	10. Medication	13. Guilty
2. Both	5. A	8. A	11. Anxiety	14. Weight
3. Both	6. D	9. Depression	12. Goodbye	

Depression

What it is

Depression is a mental disorder marked by a sad or irritable mood lasting more than two weeks.

Everyone gets sad or irritable from time to time, but for most people these moods only last for a few hours or a few days. When these feelings last for several weeks without improving, a person's way of thinking can be altered and the person may become clinically depressed.

Who gets it

About 5% of the population suffers from depression, but this number increases with age, disability, or illness. Depression is four times more likely to strike individuals over age 65 than younger people. 15% of older adults are depressed. People with disabilities or illness, and those who take care of them, have depression rates ranging from 20% to 50%.

Cause of depression

Depression has many different causes. Some causes include:

- Medication side effects, particularly from drugs used to treat arthritis, heart problems, high blood pressure, or cancer

- Illnesses such as Alzheimer's disease, Parkinson's disease, stroke, hormonal disorders, and others

- Genetics—it may run in families

- A traumatic event, such as a death in the family

- Changes or differences in brain chemistry

Signs of depression

If a person has four or more of these symptoms lasting two weeks or more, he or she may be depressed.

- Sad, depressed, or apathetic mood. May cry a lot, or complain of feeling empty.

- Irritability, agitation, grumpiness.

- Disturbed sleep—either difficulty sleeping, or sleeping more than usual.

- Fatigue and loss of energy.

- Changes in appetite and weight—either increased or decreased.

- Loss of interest or pleasure in normal activities, such as self-care or social activities.

- Withdrawal from others.

- Feelings of worthlessness, guilt, helplessness, hopelessness, or self-reproach.

- Thoughts of death or suicide, or attempted suicide.

- Difficulty thinking, concentrating, focusing, or remembering.

- Slowed or agitated movements or speech.

- Complaining of aches and pains, dizziness, blurred vision, racing heart, anxiety, or vague discomforts.

- Constant complaining.

- Mood swings.

- Excessive alcohol use.

 ## Signs of depression

To personalize this lesson and help staff members better understand depression, ask the group to share their experiences dealing with residents, friends, or family who were depressed. Ask them to describe common characteristics, and write answers on a flip chart.

Anxiety

What it is

Anxiety is a feeling of concern or worry, and includes increased alertness or awareness. It can be mild, moderate, or severe; when very severe it can become a state of panic.

Mild to moderate anxiety is a normal part of living, and can even be helpful when we must focus on something urgent or important. As a normal reaction to a stressful situation, it helps us take action. When anxiety becomes a long-term condition, or becomes severe, the person becomes overly focused on specific details and can't think of anything else. In this case, most of the individual's behavior is directed toward relieving the anxiety.

Who gets it

From 3% to 8% of the population have severe anxiety, with about 15% of people experiencing it at some point in their lives. It is a very common disorder in the elderly, and is more common in women than men.

Causes

Some of the many causes of anxiety are:

- Persistent stress

- Extreme change

- Illness, particularly cancer, heart disease, and chronic illnesses

- Chemical changes in the brain

- Abnormal brain functioning

- Medication side effects

- Drug abuse or withdrawal

Signs of anxiety

There are five main types of severe anxiety, and each has different symptoms.

- **Generalized anxiety disorder:** This condition involves excessive and unreasonable anxiety and worry lasting at last six months. Signs include restlessness, fatigue, difficulty concentrating, irritability, muscle tension, shaking, crying, pacing, sweating, rapid breathing, rapid heartbeat, fearfulness, and sleep problems.

- **Panic disorder:** People with this condition have recurring attacks of panic. They may have dizziness, faint feelings, sweating, trembling, chills, flushes, nausea, numbness, heart palpitations, or chest pain. These attacks occur suddenly and last several minutes.

- **Obsessive-compulsive disorder:** This disorder causes recurrent and persistent thoughts, impulses, or images that are unwanted and inappropriate. The person performs repetitive behaviors in response to these thoughts.

- **Phobias:** These are irrational, intense fears of certain things or situations, that interfere with normal functioning.

- **Post-traumatic stress disorder:** This occurs after a person experiences or witnesses a traumatic event. Symptoms include recurring memories, nightmares, and flashbacks.

Signs of depression

To personalize this lesson and help staff members better understand depression, ask the group to share their experiences dealing with residents, friends, or family who were depressed. Ask them to describe common characteristics, and write answers on a flip chart.

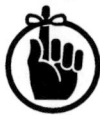

Even though depression and anxiety are common, they are NOT normal, even among the disabled, ill, or elderly. These signs should always be reported to a physician. Other diseases can cause some of these symptoms, so the doctor will have to decide on a diagnosis and a treatment. We must never assume that these signs are a normal part of disability, illness, or aging.

Preventing depression and anxiety

Although many types of depression and anxiety cannot be prevented, there are some general things that everyone can do to lower the risk of developing these conditions.

1. Keep and maintain friendships and social activities.

2. Develop enjoyable interests or hobbies.

3. Stay physically active. Exercise and stay physically fit.

4. Stay mentally active. Read, take classes, and learn new things.

5. Maintain contact with family members.

6. Eat a balanced and nutritious diet. Avoid sugar, caffeine, and alcohol.

7. Follow the doctor's directions on using the medicines to lower the risk of those side effects.

Caring for people with depression and anxiety

Depression

- Encourage depressed people to express their feelings. Listen to what they say. Accept them as they are without making judgments. Give them time to get their thoughts together and to tell you what they are thinking and feeling. Help them feel valued.

- Brighten the environment by hanging pictures, posters, or family photos. Make family photo albums easily available. Keep the environment neat and clean.

- Encourage pleasant activities such as listening to music or performing a hobby.

- Encourage socialization. Start with one-to-one conversations, and gradually help residents participate in larger social events.

- Encourage daily exercise or activity. Even the disabled can usually move a few body parts.

- Encourage as much self-care as possible. Help the person gain a sense of control by letting him or her make as many independent decisions as possible.

- Pay attention if someone talks of self-injury or suicide. Always report this to a supervisor.

- Be sure the person takes his or her medications in the correct way and at the correct time.

Anxiety

- Listen to a person's fears and anxieties. Respond with reassurance and support.

- The environment should be quiet and less stimulating than normal.

- Many people will never become completely free from anxiety. Help them learn to accept and tolerate a certain level of worry and anxiety. If they believe that you will assist them with their problems and keep them safe, their anxiety may be relieved.

- Sometimes an anxious person can be distracted if you help him or her think about something pleasant or relaxing, or have him or her picture a peaceful image.

- Help the person relax each muscle, guiding him or her to consciously and progressively relax every muscle from toes to head. Instruct him or her to breathe slowly and deeply.

- Help anxious people recognize that although their feelings are real, their fears are not based on reality. Gently point this out: "You're feeling anxious, but you are really okay."

- Ensure that medications are taken as prescribed.

The warning signs of suicide

Sometimes anxiety and depression occur together, or one may lead to the other. People suffering from either one of these illnesses may decide they want to end their life. It is important to be alert to things that might indicate a person is seriously considering suicide. The suicide rate is twice as high in people over age 65 as it is in younger age groups. Untreated or mistreated depression can lead to suicide. Pay attention to these warning signs and report them.

Pass out and discuss the "signs of suicide" handout.

Signs of suicide

✔ Talking about suicide. Statements such as "I have no reason to go on living" are danger signs.

✔ Being preoccupied with death.

✔ Giving things away.

✔ Stockpiling pills or obtaining some sort of weapon.

✔ Refusing to follow doctor's orders about medications or diet.

✔ Making unusual visits or calls to family and friends, saying goodbye to loved ones.

✔ Getting affairs in order or making funeral arrangements.

✔ Losing interest in things or people that used to be important.

✔ Suddenly becoming happier and calmer after a period of depression or anxiety.

✔ Talking about how worthless or helpless they are, saying they have no hopes or plans.

 Also appears on your CD-ROM.

Suicide prevention

Here are some things you can do to help prevent someone from taking his or her own life:

1. Recognize anxiety and depression in others and help them get appropriate treatment.

2. Remove any weapons and be sure the environment is safe and secure.

3. If you suspect someone is thinking about suicide, ask them if they are. Don't be afraid that you'll be giving them ideas. If they tell you they are having these thoughts, report it.

4. Be sure a depressed or anxious person is seeing the doctor as ordered and getting their medications.

5. Reassure a suicidal person of how much you care. Explain that depression is no one's fault, that it can be treated, and that suicidal thoughts are temporary and will go away.

6. Don't try to minimize the individual's problems. Don't tell the person how hurt his or her family will be or that he or she has everything to live for, because this just makes the person feel guilty and even more hopeless.

7. If you suspect someone is thinking about suicide, always report your suspicions to the appropriate person. Don't think that you are imagining things or getting worried for nothing. It is much better to be cautious in this situation.

If one of your residents or patients shows warning signs of suicide, contact your supervisor immediately—time could be very important.

People commit suicide because they think it is the only way to stop the pain they are feeling. Our job is to help them find other ways to get rid of their pain, through appropriate care and treatment.

QUIZ

Depression and anxiety

Name: _____

Date: _____ **Score:** _____

Here is a list of things that can be done to help people with depression or anxiety. Beside the items that are helpful in Depression, write a "D." Beside the items that are helpful in Anxiety, write an "A." If the item is helpful to both disorders, write "Both."

_____ 1. Keep the environment bright and clean.

_____ 2. Listen.

_____ 3. Encourage daily exercise.

_____ 4. Help the person breathe deeply and relax their muscles.

_____ 5. Reassure the person that you will help them and keep them safe.

_____ 6. Encourage the individual to be with people and participate in social events.

_____ 7. Make sure medications are given as ordered.

_____ 8. Keep the environment quiet and nonstimulating.

Fill in the blanks in the statements below:

9. A person who feels unneeded or unwanted may be suffering from _____.

10. Illness, chemical changes in the brain, and _____ side effects can all cause depression or anxiety.

11. Someone who is constantly fearful or restless may be suffering from _____.

12. Saying _____ to loved ones could be a sign that a person is thinking about suicide.

13. Telling a suicidal person that he will hurt his family if he kills himself only makes him feel more hopeless and _____, thereby increasing his pain.

14. Losing or gaining _____ could be a sign of depression.

 Also appears on your CD-ROM.

CERTIFICATE OF COMPLETION

This is to certify that

_____

has read and successfully passed the final exam of

Depression and anxiety

_____

Supervisor name

Diabetes

Overview

This lesson is designed to help workers understand diabetes.

Program time

Approximately 45 minutes

Learning objectives

After completing this lesson, participants will be able to do the following:

- Explain what diabetes is and does

- Describe the four key elements of treatment for diabetes

- List the symptoms of low blood sugar and high blood sugar

- Know how to respond to a diabetic emergency

Preparation

1. Familiarize yourself with the information by reviewing the lesson prior to teaching it.

2. Print and pass out appropriate handout(s) when instructed.

3. Print out a quiz and certificate for each learner from the CD-ROM.

Method

1. Deliver a mini-lecture covering the material in the workbook on pages 15–22. To make teaching easier, use the instruction icons as cues for leading the session. Be sure to insert your facility's policies and procedures whenever appropriate.

2. Encourage participant discussion when appropriate.

3. Hand out the quiz and allow adequate time for each participant to finish.

4. Give certificates of completion to those who correctly answered at least seven of the questions.

Answer key

1. 80–130; 100–150	3. B	6. 70	9. True
2. Diet, exercise,	4. False	7. 180	10. Feet, skin
medication, monitoring	5. True	8. False	11. True

Diabetes

What it is

Diabetes is a disease that changes the way our bodies use food. It causes the level of sugar in the blood to be too high. The extra sugar harms the blood vessels and other organs in the body over time. Diabetes can cause great damage before any symptoms appear.

When we eat, our bodies digest the food and turn it into sugar, or glucose. In a normal healthy person, an organ called the pancreas produces insulin, a hormone. Insulin helps the body's cells use glucose to produce energy. The cells use this energy to keep our bodies healthy.

In someone with diabetes, either the pancreas is not producing enough insulin or the body does not use its insulin effectively. The cells cannot turn sugar into energy, and the sugar builds up in the blood. The cells are starved for energy, and the blood carries dangerously high levels of sugar that can't be used.

The two main types of diabetes

Type 1

Type 1 means that the pancreas is not producing insulin, or is producing very little. This type always requires shots of insulin injected into the body every day. This form of diabetes usually strikes children and young adults, although disease onset can occur at any age. Type 1 diabetes may account for 5% to 10% of all diagnosed cases of diabetes.

Type 2

Type 2 means that the pancreas is producing insulin, but not enough, or that the body does not use its insulin effectively.

Nine out of 10 cases of diabetes are Type 2. It usually occurs in people over age 45 who are overweight. It can be treated by diet, exercise, and/or medications that are taken by mouth. Sometimes it also requires insulin injections.

Why is it important to control diabetes?

The goal of treatment for diabetes is to keep the individual's blood sugar as close to normal as possible for that person. Doing this will lower the person's chances of getting:

- Stroke
- Heart disease
- Kidney failure
- Stomach disease
- High blood pressure
- Eye disease, loss of vision, or blindness
- Nerve damage, with pain or loss of feeling in hands, feet, legs, or other parts of the body

A high level of sugar in the blood over a long period of time causes these problems.

Four parts to diabetic treatment

There are four main parts to treating diabetes:

1. Diet

2. Exercise

3. Medication

4. Monitoring

Diet

There is no one diabetic diet designed for every diabetic person. There are guidelines to help diabetics with food choices. These guidelines are very similar to the kind of eating that is healthy for anyone. These are the main rules that should be followed:

1. Eat few sugary foods.

2. Eat less fat, especially saturated fat and cholesterol (butter, margarine, oils).

3. Eat a variety of fresh fruits, vegetables, lean meats, and fish.

4. Eat just enough calories to maintain a healthy weight.

Diabetics should eat the recommended number of servings from all the food groups on this pyramid every day, except for the fats, sweets, and alcohol. No one needs sweets or alcohol for good nutrition (they can be an occasional treat), and we get plenty of fats from the other food groups. The exact number of servings a diabetic should have from each group depends on individual calorie and nutrition needs, weight goals, exercise level, and preferences.

Diabetics and sugar

Many people think that diabetics are not allowed to eat sugar of any kind. This is no longer required. Sugar is a carbohydrate, like bread or potatoes, and can be part of the diabetic's food plan. However, most sugary foods provide calories without many vitamins or minerals, and they are often high in fat. It is better to eat more foods rich in nutrients, like vegetables and fruits, and very few fatty, sweet foods like ice cream and candy.

Dietitians sometimes teach diabetics and those who care for them to use Exchange Lists. These lists are a way to plan meals by putting foods in a category, such as a starch exchange or fruit exchange. Foods on a list can be substituted for each other and sometimes for foods on other exchange lists. The diabetic person eats only a certain number of each type of exchange every day, as ordered by a doctor or established by the dietitian.

Exercise

Exercise usually lowers blood sugar and may help insulin work better. It helps control weight, it improves blood flow, and it strengthens the heart. People with diabetes should exercise at least three times a week. Before a diabetic starts a new exercise program, a doctor should approve what kind, how often, and how long the diabetic exercises. Elderly and disabled people need to exercise also, and should be helped to find an exercise they can do.

It is important that a diabetic not develop low blood sugar while exercising. Since the body burns sugar during exercise, the diabetic should "fuel up" with a piece of fruit or half a sandwich within an hour before starting any exercise. It is also a good idea for the diabetic to check his or her blood sugar level before he or she starts exercising. If the blood sugar reading is less than 70, he or she should eat something and wait for the blood sugar level to come up over 70 before exercising.

If a diabetic feels faint, sweaty, dizzy, or confused while doing any activity, he or she should stop what he or she is doing and immediately drink fruit juice or a sweet (not diet) soft drink. He or she must respond quickly to this feeling, because it means his or her blood sugar level is too low.

Medication

Diabetics might receive insulin shots or they may take pills by mouth. Only a doctor can decide what medication and how much of it a diabetic should receive. It can be VERY dangerous to change a diabetic's medication in any way unless it is ordered by a doctor. Diabetics must receive the exact amount of medicine their doctor has ordered, at the times the doctor has ordered. Timing of medicine and meals is important to prevent low blood sugar.

Monitoring

Close monitoring of a diabetic's blood sugar level is one of the best ways for him or her to prevent long-term complications from the disease. Diabetics check their blood sugar by pricking a finger with a needle and testing a drop of blood with a special blood glucose meter. The meter, also called a monitor, gives a number that tells the level of glucose in the blood. These monitors must be kept clean and should be checked for accuracy periodically.

Most diabetics need their blood sugar level tested at least once a day, usually in the morning before breakfast. Depending on the type of diabetes, the age of the person, and other factors, the individual may need his or her blood glucose tested as much as five times a day. Sometimes insulin dosages are adjusted depending on the blood sugar level. This chart from the National Diabetes Education Program shows the recommended blood sugar levels at different times of the day:

Before meals	80–130
At bedtime	100–150

A doctor must set the acceptable ranges **for each person,** and **they might differ from the normal ranges** given in the chart. When a blood glucose level falls outside the range set by the doctor, the doctor must be notified as soon as possible. If you are assisting a diabetic with monitoring his or her blood sugar, be sure you know the correct range for that person.

Another important part of monitoring is watching the feet and skin of a diabetic. Diabetes can turn a small sore or wound into a very large problem. Sores, blisters, and wounds on a resident's feet and skin must always be reported to your supervisor or a nurse.

Diabetic emergencies and how to respond

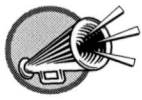 *Diabetes can cause both long-term and short-term problems. Blood sugar that is too low or extremely high can lead rapidly to unconsciousness and even death. You must know the symptoms of both conditions and know how to respond.*

Hypoglycemia

Hypoglycemia means that the level of sugar in the blood is too low (less than 70). Too much insulin or oral medication, too much exercise, not eating enough food, or drinking alcohol can cause it. Hypoglycemia can cause strokes and heart attacks in the elderly. This problem is also called insulin reaction or insulin shock.

Symptoms of low blood sugar

These symptoms can appear suddenly and without warning:

- Shaky, nervous

- Sweaty and cold

- Pale, clammy skin

- Weak and tired, drowsy

- Sudden hunger

- Blurred or double vision

- Tingling of hands, lips, or tongue

- Confusion

- Personality change

- Slurred speech

- Loss of consciousness

- Dizziness, or a staggering walk

- Nausea

- Headache

- Fast heartbeat

- Itching

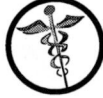 *Elderly people and people with other diseases and disabilities can be especially sensitive to low blood sugar, and it can be very dangerous for them. Some people may have a reaction even when their blood sugar is not below 70. Any diabetic suddenly showing any of the signs listed above must receive* **immediate** *attention.*

Treatment

If you suspect that a resident is suffering from hypoglycemia, talk to your supervisor immediately. Treatment can include:

- Drinking a sweet drink such as sweetened coffee or tea, orange juice, or soda

- Eating sugar, corn syrup, or candy, or taking glucose tablets

Hyperglycemia

Hyperglycemia means that the level of sugar in the blood is too high (above 180). It can be caused by infections, illness, stress, injury, not enough insulin, not enough exercise, or eating too much food. Very high levels of sugar can cause coma and death.

Symptoms of high blood sugar

These symptoms occur gradually and get worse over time:

- Extreme thirst and/or hunger

- Rapid weight loss

- Frequent urination

- Vision changes

- Dry skin and mouth

- Fatigue and drowsiness

- Nausea

- Fruity-smelling breath

- Very deep, gasping breathing

Treatment

If you notice any of these symptoms, notify your supervisor or a nurse as soon as possible. Fruity-smelling breath, deep gasping breathing, and unconsciousness are emergency symptoms that can lead quickly to death. Call 911 or access emergency medical care at once.

Case studies

The following case studies are examples of things that sometimes happen in nursing homes. Have students pair up and write answers for each case study in their workbooks. After each pair has had sufficient time to answer each, discuss answers with the entire class.

Case study #1

Mrs. Jarvis is diabetic. One day as you are assisting her with her shower, you notice that she seems confused. She doesn't seem to understand what you say to her, and she acts nervous. Her skin feels cool and damp and looks paler than usual.

What do you think might be happening to Mrs. Jarvis? What, if anything, should you do?

Answer:

Mrs. Jarvis is probably suffering from low blood sugar. She should be given a drink of fruit juice or other sweetened drink (tea or coffee with sugar, nondiet soda), or assisted to take some sugar cubes or glucose tablets. If possible, her blood sugar should be checked.

If Mrs. Jarvis does not get better or gets worse, or if her blood sugar is outside her approved range and does not improve when rechecked, medical assistance should be summoned.

Case study #2

One morning Mr. Young's blood sugar reading is 250. He seems fine and says he feels great. Mr. Young's doctor said his blood sugar should not go above 220.

What should you do in this situation?

Answer:

Mr. Young's blood sugar is too high and must be reported to his physician. Even though he has no symptoms, this condition could worsen without treatment. In addition, a blood sugar this high is causing hidden long-term problems in his body. Follow your facility's protocol for notifying your supervisor, a nurse, or the doctor.

Case study #3

Mrs. Bond checks her blood sugar and gives herself insulin every morning. You are supposed to remind her to do this. When you remind her, she always tells you that she has done it or is about to do it. Lately you've noticed that Mrs. Bond seems to be losing weight. You watch to be sure she is eating, and you see that she is eating a large amount of food. She has starting urinating on herself sometimes, and when you help her get cleaned up she says that she is urinating a lot and sometimes she just can't make it to the bathroom. When you suggest that she should cut back on the water she is drinking, she tells you that she is thirsty all the time.

What is going on with Mrs. Bond? What action, if any, should you take?

Answer:

Mrs. Bond might have an inaccurate glucose monitor machine, she might not be taking her insulin correctly, or she might be forgetting to take it in spite of your reminders. Her symptoms indicate that her blood sugar is too high. Her blood sugar should be checked. Even if her blood sugar is normal, these symptoms must be reported to her doctor.

QUIZ

Diabetes

Name: _____

Date: _____ Score: _____

Circle or write the correct answer.

1. Fill in the chart of normal recommended blood sugar levels with the missing numbers: (Worth two points)

Before Meals	
At Bedtime	

2. Write the four parts of diabetic treatment: (Worth four points)
    a. _____ b. _____ c. _____ d. _____

3. If a diabetic person becomes weak, tired, and dizzy, you should first: (circle one)
    a. Have her lie down until it wears off.
    b. Give her something sweet to drink.
    c. Call 911.

4. Diabetics should never eat candy, ice cream, or cake.
    True   or   False   (circle one)

5. Having high levels of sugar in the blood over a long period of time can cause heart disease, blindness, and loss of feeling in the feet.
    True   or   False   (circle one)

6. For most people, blood sugar is too low if it reads less than _____ on a glucose meter.

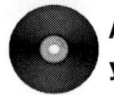 **Also appears on your CD-ROM.**

QUIZ

Diabetes (cont.)

7. For most people, blood sugar is too high if it reads more than _____ on a glucose meter.

8. All diabetics must take insulin shots.
   True   or   False   (circle one)

9. All diabetics should monitor their blood sugar, control their diet, exercise, and take their medicines.
   True   or   False   (circle one)

10. If you notice sores or wounds on the _____ or _____ of a diabetic, you must report them to your supervisor or a medical person. (Worth two points)

11. Low blood sugar can cause heart attacks and strokes in the elderly.
    True   or   False   (circle one)

CERTIFICATE OF COMPLETION

This is to certify that

_____

has read and successfully passed the final exam of

Diabetes

_____

Supervisor name

Incontinence

Overview

This lesson is designed to help workers understand and recognize the signs of incontinence.

Program time

Approximately 45 minutes

Learning objectives

After completing this lesson, participants will be able to do the following:

- Know the causes of common urinary and bowel elimination problems

- Be able to state the best ways to help residents with these problems

- Understand various behavioral, nutritional, and care interventions for urinary and bowel incontinence and constipation

Preparation

1. Familiarize yourself with the information by reviewing the lesson prior to teaching it.

2. Print and pass out appropriate handout(s) when instructed.

3. Print out a quiz and certificate for each learner from the CD-ROM.

Method

1. Deliver a mini-lecture covering the material in the workbook on pages 23–29. To make teaching easier, use the instruction icons as cues for leading the session. Be sure to insert your facility's policies and procedures whenever appropriate.

2. Encourage participant discussion when appropriate.

3. Hand out the quiz and allow adequate time for each participant to finish.

4. Give certificates of completion to those who correctly answered at least seven of the questions.

Answer key

1. A	2. C	3. B	4. C	5. False	6. False	7. True
8. True	9. C	10. True	11. False	12. True		

Incontinence

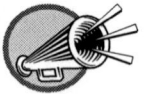 *Ask your learners, "How many of you think that being unable to control your bladder or your bowels is a normal part of aging?" This is a common misconception, and it is likely that many of your learners will agree that your statement is true. Then ask, "Do you think anything can be done to improve the problem in older people?" Many times we just accept there is nothing that can be done for these conditions except to wear protective clothing. Often difficulty with controlling the bladder or bowels leads to the decision to enter a care facility. However, there are things that can be done by caregivers that can help control these problems, thereby improving the resident's quality of life.*

People who cannot control when or where they urinate suffer from urinary incontinence, or U.I. There are things that can be done to improve this condition, but it is important to know what the *cause* is so the right care and treatment can be given. This condition is not the person's fault, and it is not a necessary or normal part of growing older. It is not caused by laziness or meanness. U.I. is a health problem with a number of possible causes.

Some of the most common causes include:

- Urinary tract infections

- Confusion and forgetfulness

- Muscle weakness

- Vaginal problems (women)

- Prostate problems (men)

- Medication reactions

- Problems with clothing

- Trouble getting to the bathroom

- Constipation

Symptoms

Any resident who ever wets the bed or himself, leaks urine on the way to the bathroom, or has to use protective pads or padded briefs is suffering from UI. If you notice a resident, a bed, or a room that has urine stains or a urine odor, then you know the resident needs help with this condition. However, you probably don't know what kind of UI the resident might have. You can often determine this by watching the resident closely and keeping track of his or her urinating habits on a bladder record. It shows regular daily habits as well as accidents. Keeping a *bladder record* is an excellent way to get information about a resident's UI so ways can be found to treat it.

Pass out the Bladder Record handout and explain how it can be used at your facility.

Sample bladder record

Name: _____ **Date:** _____

Instructions: Place a check in the appropriate column next to the time you urinated in the toilet or when an incontinence episode occurred. Note the reason for the incontinence and describe your liquid intake (for example, coffee, water) and estimate the amount (for example, one cup).

Time interval	Urinated in toilet	Had a small incontinence episode	Had a large incontinence episode	Reason for incontinence episode	Type/amount of liquid intake
6 - 8 a.m.					
8 - 10 a.m.					
10 - noon					
Noon - 2 p.m.					
2 - 4 p.m.					
4 - 6 p.m.					
6 - 8 p.m.					
8 - 10 p.m.					
10 - midnight					
Overnight					
No. of pads used today:			No. of pads used today:		

Comments: _____

Also appears on your CD-ROM.

There are three different types of U.I.:

- With urge incontinence, people may leak urine on their way to the bathroom, after they drink just a little bit of liquid, or as soon as they feel the urge to go.

- Stress incontinence may cause urine to leak when they sneeze, cough, or laugh, or when they exercise or move a certain way (getting out of bed, up from a chair, walking, lifting). This is common in women.

- Overflow incontinence causes people to feel they need to urinate again right after going, or to feel as though they never totally empty the bladder, or to pass small amounts of urine without feeling any need to go. It may be a sign of prostate problems in men.

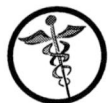

Helping residents with urinary incontinence

Your first responsibility is to report U.I. to your supervisor, the facility nurse, or the resident's doctor. A doctor or nurse should check a resident with U.I., and your observations about the resident, such as a bladder record, will help him or her determine the cause and type of U.I.

The three treatments for U.I. are:

1. Medicine.

2. Surgery.

3. Behavioral treatments. These help people control their urine and use the toilet at the right time. They work well for residents who have problems getting to the bathroom or who are not able to tell you when they need to urinate. Three behavioral interventions that you can help with include:

    - Scheduled toileting

    - Prompted voiding

    - Habit training

Scheduled toileting

Use scheduled toileting for residents who can't get out of bed or can't get to the bathroom alone. To do this treatment, assist the resident to the bathroom every two to four hours on a regular schedule.

Prompted voiding

Use prompted voiding for residents who know when they have a full bladder, but do not ask to go to the bathroom. To do this treatment:

1. Check the resident often for wetness.

2. Ask, "Do you want to use the toilet?"

3. Help the resident to the toilet.

4. Praise the resident for being dry.

5. Tell the resident when you will come back to take him or her to the bathroom again.

Habit training

Use habit training for residents who tend to urinate at about the same time every day. To do this:

1. Watch the resident to find what times he or she urinates. A bladder record can help you do this.

2. Take the resident to the bathroom at those times every day.

3. Praise the resident for being dry and using the toilet.

For all behavioral treatments

1. Be patient. These treatments take time.

2. Treat the resident as an adult.

3. Answer a call bell as soon as possible.

4. Do not rush the resident.

5. Give the resident plenty of time to completely empty his or her bladder.

6. Give privacy by closing the door, even if you must stay in the bathroom.

7. **Never** yell or be angry with the resident if he or she is wet. Say, "You can try again next time."

8. Respect dignity and confidentiality.

Other ways to help residents with U.I.

1. Pelvic exercises can make muscles around the bladder stronger and help with U.I. These are called Kegel exercises, and to do them the person tightens the pelvic muscles that stop and start the flow of urine. The muscles should be squeezed tightly for a few seconds and then released, up to 10 times at one sitting, four times every day. Then, whenever the person feels that urine might leak, he or she tightens those same muscles and prevents urine from leaking.

2. People who can't get out of bed or can't get to the bathroom for some reason may need to use a bedpan, urinal, or bedside commode. These articles, if needed, should be kept by the bed.

3. If a resident uses a wheelchair, walker, or cane to get to the bathroom, you can help by keeping the item near the bed, keeping the path to the bathroom clear and well lit, and answering calls for assistance as soon as possible.

4. Encourage the resident to wear clothes that are easy to remove and have simple fasteners.

5. If a resident needs to wear special pads or clothing to help keep the skin dry, these should be changed often. Use soft pads and clothing, keep them wrinkle-free, keep the skin clean and dry, and use protective skin creams if allowed. Remember that wet skin can develop sores and rashes.

6. If the resident wets the bed at night, it might be helpful to restrict evening liquids, but you should only do this if a doctor or nurse orders it. This is usually done in the three hours before bedtime. The resident should use the bathroom just before going to bed.

7. Some residents need to use a urinary catheter, which is a tube inserted into the bladder by a doctor or nurse. It drains urine into a bag. Sometimes men use a condom catheter that fits over the penis. Catheters can cause infections, and condom catheters that are too tight can be harmful. Catheters should be checked often. They are not recommended for most incontinence problems.

Bowel incontinence

People who cannot control when or where they pass gas or stool suffer from bowel incontinence. There are things that can be done to improve this condition, but it is important to know what the cause is so the right care and treatment can be given. This condition is not the person's fault, and it is not a necessary part of growing older. It is a health problem that is not caused by laziness or bad behavior.

Causes

Some of the most common causes include:

- Incorrect diet or fluid intake

- Confusion and forgetfulness

- Muscle injury or weakness (the anal muscles)

- Nerve injury

- Medication reactions or laxative abuse

- Trouble getting to the bathroom

- Constipation or impaction

- Diarrhea

Helping residents with bowel incontinence

Your first responsibility is to report episodes of bowel incontinence to your supervisor, the facility nurse, or the resident's doctor. A doctor or nurse should check the resident, and your observations may help them determine the cause of the problem.

Treatments for bowel incontinence include:

1. Medicine

2. Surgery

3. Dietary management

4. Bowel management and retraining

5. Biofeedback

Two of these treatments involve the care you provide: diet management and bowel retraining. These treatments are the same as those used to help people with constipation.

Constipation

People usually say they are constipated when they are having infrequent bowel movements, but constipation is also used to refer to a sense of bloating or intestinal fullness, a decrease in the amount of stool, the need to strain to have a bowel movement, or the need to use laxatives, suppositories, or enemas to maintain regular bowel movements. It is normal for most people to have bowel movements anywhere from three times a day to three times a week, but some people may go a week or longer without discomfort or harmful effects.

Many things can cause constipation, but the most common causes include:

- Inadequate fiber and fluid intake

- Inactivity or a sedentary lifestyle

- Change in routine

- Abnormal growths or diseases

- Damaged or injured muscles (sometimes from repeatedly ignoring the urge to go)

- Medication side effects and laxative abuse

Helping residents with constipation

Your first responsibility is to report a resident's constipation problems to your supervisor, the facility nurse, or the resident's doctor. A doctor or nurse should check the resident, and your observations may help them determine the cause of the problem.

Treatments for constipation include:

1. Medicine

2. Surgery

3. Dietary management

4. Bowel management and retraining, with establishment of a habit regimen

Two of these treatments involve the care you provide: diet management and bowel retraining. These treatments are the same as those used to help people with bowel incontinence.

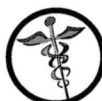

Dietary management for U.I.

While there is no dietary treatment for urinary incontinence, some foods and drinks can irritate the bladder, such as sugar, chocolate, citrus fruits (oranges, grapefruits, lemons, limes), alcohol, grape juice, and caffeinated drinks like coffee, tea, and cola. Residents with U.I. could try eliminating these foods and beverages from their diet and see if the condition improves.

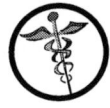

Dietary management for bowel incontinence and constipation

The average American diet contains 10 to 15 grams of fiber a day. The amount of fiber recommended for good bowel function is **25 to 30 grams of fiber per day,** plus 60 to 80 ounces of fluid. Look at the table below to get an idea of the fiber we get in different foods. Most people can successfully treat their bowel irregularities, both incontinence and constipation, by adding high-fiber foods to their diets, along with increasing fluid intake to desired levels. Increase dietary fiber slowly to give the bowel time to adjust. **People with diverticulosis or diverticulitis should not consume a high-fiber diet.**

Fiber	Fiber grams	Higher-fiber alternatives	Fiber grams
Breads White bread, 1 slice	0.50	Whole wheat bread, 1 slice	2.11
Cereals Corn flakes, 1 oz.	0.45	Oat bran cereal, 1 oz.	4.06
Rice White rice, ½ cup	1.42	Brown rice, ½ cup	5.27
Vegetables Lettuce, ½ cup raw	0.24	Green peas, ½ cup	3.36
Beans Green beans, ½ cup	1.89	Pinto beans, ½ cup	5.93
Fresh Fruits Banana, 1 medium	2.19	Blackberries, 1 cup	7.20

Food sensitivities: Some people are sensitive to, or even allergic to, certain foods that cause them constipation or diarrhea. Dairy products such as milk and cheese, wheat products such as bread, and foods containing chocolate are some of the more common problem foods. A physician should evaluate a resident who seems to have particular food sensitivities.

QUIZ

Incontinence

Name: _____

Date: _____ Score: _____

Circle or write the correct answers.

1. **What are some causes of both bowel and urinary incontinence?**
   a. Muscle weakness, confusion, or medication reactions
   b. Laziness, poor manners, or meanness
   c. Stupidity, uncooperativeness, and sloppiness

2. **Scheduled toileting, prompted voiding, and habit training are:**
   a. Not encouraged by physicians, nurses, or state regulations
   b. Responsibilities of the nurse or facility manager, not the attendant
   c. Recommended behavioral treatments for urinary incontinence
   d. Too time-consuming to be practical

3. **For the best bowel function, we should consume how much dietary fiber every day?**
   a. 10 to 15 grams
   b. 25 to 30 grams
   c. 45 to 50 grams

4. **Kegel exercises are done by:**
   a. Circling the ankles around and around and then up and down
   b. Lowering the chin to the chest, then turning the head side to side
   c. Tightening the pelvic muscles that control the flow of urine

5. **Urinary catheters are often recommended to treat urinary incontinence.**
   True   False

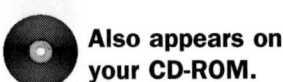

**Also appears on
your CD-ROM.**

QUIZ

Incontinence (cont.)

6. **Bowel retraining and behavioral treatments for urinary incontinence usually work quickly, fixing the problem within a week or less.**
   True   False

7. **Most fruits and beans contain higher dietary fiber than white breads and rice.**
   True   False

8. **It is important to keep residents with urinary or bowel incontinence clean and dry so their skin is protected from developing sores.**
   True   False

9. **Habit training can be used to help both urinary and bowel incontinence. It consists of:**
   a. Assisting the resident to the bathroom every two to four hours.
   b. Checking the resident often and asking him if he wants to use the bathroom.
   c. Assisting the resident to the bathroom at scheduled times every day.
   d. Writing the resident's habits down on a form

10. **Stress incontinence might cause urine to leak when someone sneezes or laughs.**
    True   False

11. **A person who has a bowel movement only three or four times a week is constipated.**
    True   False

12. **A resident with incontinence should be treated as an adult, with dignity.**
    True   False

CERTIFICATE OF COMPLETION

This is to certify that

_____

has read and successfully passed the final exam of

Incontinence

_____

Supervisor name

Malnutrition and dehydration

Overview

This lesson is designed to help workers understand and recognize the signs and symptoms of malnutrition and dehydration.

Program time
Approximately 45 minutes

Learning objectives
After completing this lesson, participants will be able to do the following:

- Explain physical and chemical changes in the ill and elderly that affect the way their bodies absorb nutrients from food

- Explain why the body needs fluids

- Recognize symptoms that may be caused by not getting enough nutrients or fluids

- Describe foods, nutrients, and fluids that are needed every day

- Describe ways to encourage healthful eating and drinking

Preparation

1. Familiarize yourself with the information by reviewing the lesson prior to teaching it.

2. Print and pass out appropriate handout(s) when instructed.

3. Print out a quiz and certificate for each learner from the CD-ROM.

Method

1. Deliver a mini-lecture covering the material in the workbook on pages 31–38. To make teaching easier, use the instruction icons as cues for leading the session. Be sure to insert your facility's policies and procedures whenever appropriate.

2. Encourage participant discussion when appropriate.

3. Hand out the quiz and allow adequate time for each participant to finish.

4. Give certificates of completion to those who correctly answered at least seven of the questions.

Answer key

1. True	2. False	3. True	4. True	5. True	6. False
7. True	8. True	9. True	10. False		

Physical and chemical changes that influence nutritional needs

People who are sick or elderly have different food requirements than young, healthy people. They are also more likely to suffer harm from not eating the right foods. After age fifty there are chemical and physical changes in the body that affect nutritional needs.

- The metabolic rate, or metabolism, slows down. The metabolic rate is the speed at which the body uses energy. Older bodies burn less fuel for daily operations. This means seniors need fewer calories for normal everyday activities. This also applies to anyone who is not very active or is confined to bed.

- Lean tissue and muscle mass decrease. There is less bone mass. Body fat increases.

- Stomach acid may decrease and the stomach might not empty as fast. The intestine may absorb less nutrition from the food it gets.

- Tooth and gum problems increase, sometimes making it difficult to chew.

- Some people have trouble swallowing, especially those who have had strokes.

- There is a loss of taste and smell. This causes people to be less interested in food.

- Sometimes people are too tired or weak to eat an entire meal.

- Appetite and thirst decrease. Many elderly or ill people eat and drink less than they should. This leads to fatigue, sadness, infections, skin breakdown, and lack of energy.

- Medications can affect appetite or thirst. Sometimes medicines upset the stomach or cause intestinal problems like diarrhea or constipation.

- Many diseases affect the way the body uses food or water. Someone with an illness usually needs more food and water because the body needs energy to heal. People with some conditions, however, must carefully control the amount and type of calories they take in. Diabetes is one example.

 Although the body may need fewer calories because of age or inactivity, it still needs the same amount of nutrients and fluid it always has—or more. It is important to eat foods that have a high nutritional value.

Malnutrition

Bodies will break down if they do not get the type and amount of fuel they need. Malnutrition means "badly nourished," another way of saying that the person isn't getting enough of the *right* nutrients the body needs to stay healthy. It can be caused by not eating enough nutritious foods or by not adequately digesting and absorbing nutrients from food.

Getting *too much* food is harmful and is also called malnutrition.

Someone who does or experiences one or more of these things might be headed for malnutrition:

- Doesn't eat from the major food groups most of the time.

- Eats less than half of two or more meals a day.

- Eats less than one hot meal a day.

- Changes from solid foods to pureed foods, or makes other dietary changes.

- Drinks a lot of alcohol.

- Is socially isolated or depressed.

- Is poor, or has difficulty obtaining or preparing food because of physical or mental disabilities. Someone with cognitive problems might not remember to eat.

- Excessive laxative use (hinders digestion of nutrients by causing food to pass through the intestines too quickly).

- Recent surgery or illness, or chronic or multiple diseases.

Signs and symptoms of malnutrition

If a person shows any of these signs, they should be seen by a doctor. Taking care of someone with malnutrition means helping them get enough of the right nutrients.

- Tiredness and lack of energy

- Loss of appetite

- Loss of or gain in weight

- Sore lips, tongue, or throat

- Infections or slow healing

- Diarrhea or constipation

- Easy bruising

- Depression or confusion

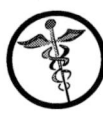 Older adults and those who are chronically ill should be weighed regularly to be sure they are getting enough calories and are not losing or gaining weight.

 Unless a person is overweight and trying to lose weight, a weight loss of just 5% of body weight can be harmful. Any *unintended* weight loss or weight gain is a sign of possible malnutrition. Report a client's changes in weight to a supervisor.

Dehydration

Dehydration is a serious, sometimes fatal condition. It means there are not enough body fluids and important blood salts in the body for it to carry on normal functions at the best level. This happens by loss of fluids, not drinking enough water, or a combination of both.

Water is essential in all the vital functions of the body. It is part of temperature regulation; building new cells; lubricating joints; and keeping the kidneys, brain, heart, and other organs working. Thirst is the warning signal that we should drink. However, just drinking when we are thirsty is not enough. Many people stay mildly dehydrated much of the time.

 You are drinking enough water if your urine is always pale in color, and you are urinating every two to three hours.

Preventing dehydration

- A healthy adult should drink at least 6–8 eight-ounce glasses of water a day.

- It is possible to get some of the necessary fluids from other drinks, but anything with caffeine in it does not count in the daily requirement. In fact, caffeinated drinks, such as coffee, tea, and cola, actually *increase* the daily requirement. Caffeine pulls water from the body, increasing the need for fluid intake. ***For every eight-ounce caffeinated drink, add an extra eight ounces of water to the daily requirement.***

- Two eight-ounce cups of coffee *increase* the daily water need to at least 8–10 eight-ounce glasses a day.

- Two twelve-ounce cans of cola *increase* the daily water need to at least 9–11 eight-ounce glasses a day.

Reasons people don't drink enough fluid

- Loss of appetite

- Lack of thirst

- Don't like frequent bathroom trips

Reasons people lose fluid

- Fever

- Vomiting

- Diarrhea

- Excessive urine output

- Excessive sweating; exercise

- Heat exhaustion

Symptoms of dehydration

Always pay attention to what clients drink and how much they urinate. The following symptoms could be signs of dehydration and must be reported immediately. Severe dehydration can result in seizures, permanent brain damage, heart and blood vessel collapse, and death if not treated quickly.

Mild dehydration

- Thirst; dry lips and tongue

- Dry membranes in the mouth

- Skin looks dry

Moderate dehydration

- Skin is not very elastic, may sag, and doesn't bounce back quickly when lightly pinched and released

- Sunken eyes

- Decreased urine output

Severe dehydration

- Small amounts of dark-colored urine

- Rapid, weak pulse over 100 (at rest)

- Rapid breathing

- Low blood pressure; dizziness

- Blue lips

- Cold hands and feet

- Confusion, lack of interest, difficult to arouse

- Shock

 Pinch a fold of skin on the back of your hand and hold it for a few seconds. Let it go, and time how quickly the skin returns to normal. The skin should return to normal within a second or two. If it stays pinched for longer than that, you may be dehydrated.

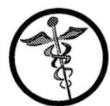

Treatment for dehydration

For mild dehydration, giving fluids by mouth is usually enough. This is called oral rehydration.

- The physician may order an oral rehydrating solution (ORS) that replaces important blood salts and water in balanced amounts designed especially for dehydration in sick people. These solutions allow the intestines to absorb maximum amounts of water.

- Don't confuse ORS with sports drinks designed for concentrated energy and salt replacement in healthy, high-performance athletes. These drinks can cause vomiting and diarrhea and are so concentrated they can limit intestinal water absorption.

- IV fluids may be necessary for moderate to severe dehydration.

- **Rapid** recognition and treatment of dehydration results in a good outcome.

A healthful, nutritious diet

Fruits and vegetables

- Everyone should eat a variety of fruits and vegetables every day.

- Different fruits and vegetables are rich in different nutrients.

- Vegetables and fruits contain fiber, vitamins, and minerals.

Grain products

- Give residents a variety of whole-grain and refined breads, cereals, pasta, and rice.

- Grains provide vitamins, minerals, carbohydrates, and fiber.

- The high fiber content of whole grains promotes proper bowel function.

Dairy

- Low-fat dairy products are needed daily to provide calcium.

- Adults over age 50 have an especially high need for calcium to maintain bone mass.

Meats and beans

- Choose from the meat and beans group each day.

- These foods provide protein to build and maintain healthy body tissues.

- People need more protein when they are dealing with illness, surgery, or trauma.

Fats

- Fats are highly concentrated sources of energy, and they provide fatty acids needed for good health.

- Monounsaturated oils (canola, olive) are believed to lower unhealthy cholesterol levels (LDL) and raise healthy cholesterol levels (HDL).

- Avoid saturated fat. Choose lean cuts of meat and remove the skin from poultry.

Water

- Water is the most important nutrient in the body. Oxygen is the only thing the body craves more.

- At least six to eight glasses of fluid are needed every day.

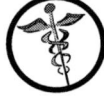

Ways to help people get needed nutrients

Care providers have a responsibility to ensure that clients' food needs are met.

- Fit the amount and the kinds of food to the individual. Serve tasty food.

- Increase fiber to help move food through the intestines and prevent constipation.

- Encourage people to eat with family and friends.

- Use a blender or food processor for those with chewing or swallowing problems.

- People with swallowing problems can choke on liquids that are too thin. A thickening agent can be added to liquids to help them drink. They may do best using a straw.

- Chop or mash meats and vegetables with a little gravy or broth.

- Use soft foods such as tuna, eggs, cheese, and peanut butter for meat substitutes.

- Small, frequent feedings and healthful snacks can encourage some people to eat. Have fruit, yogurt, or vegetables readily available.

- Adding nonfat dry milk powder to foods such as casseroles, cream soups, puddings, or gravy increases calcium and protein intake.

- Food that is served warm (not too hot or too cold) may seem tastier.

- For someone who can't eat a whole meal, try six small meals a day.

- Offer finger foods, such as sandwiches and fruits, to those who have difficulty managing utensils. Cut food into bite-sized pieces.

- No single food can supply all the nutrients in the amounts needed. The diet should include a variety of plant foods, including whole grains, fruits, and vegetables, plus protein, dairy foods, and fats.

- Combining powdered meal mixes with milk, puddings, or fruit purees bolsters the nutrient content.

- Anyone with mouth or teeth problems will benefit from soft foods like yogurt, cottage cheese, applesauce, mashed potatoes, ice cream, puddings, milkshakes, or custards.

- Clear beef or chicken broth is a good way to get warm liquids in cold weather.

- Some people may need to take vitamins and minerals in a supplement. People who get little sunlight may need vitamin D.

- Fruit juices and milk provide fluid, nutrients, and calories, but they do not fulfill the need for six to eight glasses of water a day.

- Thirst decreases with age, so encourage older people to drink fluids throughout the day. Offer water often and keep it readily available.

Pass out the Learning Activity handout to learners and have them answer the questions in groups. After all groups have finished, review and discuss the correct answers with the class. Answers: 1. D, 2. I, 3. B, 4. C, 5. E, 6. A, 7. G, 8. H, 9. F, 10. J.

Learning activity: Solve the problem

Directions: Match the situation on the below with the best solution at the bottom of the page. Put the letter of the solution in the blank next to the problem.

1. Someone who has difficulty chewing. _____

2. Someone who has difficulty swallowing. _____

3. Someone with a dry mouth and dry skin. _____

4. Someone who can't eat an entire meal at one time. _____

5. Someone who doesn't like meat. _____

6. Someone who needs more protein but not more calories. _____

7. Someone who has trouble managing a fork, knife, and spoon. _____

8. Someone who is tired, has little energy, is depressed, and is losing weight. _____

9. Someone who is confused and has sunken eyes, rapid breathing and heart rate, and small amounts of dark urine. _____

---

a. Someone who doesn't like to eat. _____

b. Add nonfat dry milk powder to foods.

c. Offer water frequently.

d. Serve six small meals a day.

e. Offer soft foods like cottage cheese; chop food into small bits.

f. Give peanut butter, cheese, eggs, and beans.

g. This person is probably seriously dehydrated. Report the person's condition to a supervisor at once.

h. Use finger foods; cut food into bite-sized pieces.

i. This person may be malnourished. Report the person's condition to a supervisor.

j. Give thickened liquids and soft foods.

k. Encourage the person to eat with friends or family. Offer frequent snacks.

 Also appears on your CD-ROM.

QUIZ

Malnutrition and Dehydration

Name: _____

Date: _____ **Score:** _____

Answer the questions by circling True or False.

1. **There is a difference in nutritional needs in the elderly compared to younger adults.** True False

2. **The elderly need fewer vitamins and minerals in their food.** True False

3. **Any weight loss or weight gain in a resident should be reported to a supervisor.** True False

4. **Protein needs increase during acute illness or surgery.** True False

5. **A diet that does not contain needed amounts of protein, vitamins, and minerals may slow the healing of a wound.** True False

6. **Someone who cannot eat enough food at a meal because of fatigue or poor appetite must wait until the next meal to eat (it is healthier to eat only three meals a day).** True False

7. **Signs of malnutrition include tiredness, weight loss, and slow healing of a wound or sore.** True False

8. **In the elderly, decreased thirst and poor intake of fluids could lead to dehydration.** True False

9. **A person whose body severely lacks fluid can suffer heart and blood vessel collapse and even death if not treated quickly.** True False

10. **When you pinch the skin on the back of someone's hand it will spring back to normal quickly if the person is dehydrated.** True False

Also appears on your CD-ROM.

CERTIFICATE OF COMPLETION

This is to certify that

_____

has read and successfully passed the final exam of

Malnutrition and dehydration

_____

Supervisor name

Elopement and wandering

Overview

This lesson is designed to help workers understand elopement and wandering behaviors.

Program time
Approximately 45 minutes

Learning objectives
After completing this lesson, participants will be able to do the following:

- Explain why people with dementia wander and elope

- Use multiple techniques to manage residents who wander and elope

- Provide a safe environment for residents who wander

- Respond appropriately to an elopement

Preparation

1. Familiarize yourself with the information by reviewing the lesson prior to teaching it.

2. Print and pass out appropriate handout(s) when instructed.

3. Print out a quiz and certificate for each learner from the CD-ROM.

Method

1. Deliver a mini-lecture covering the material in the workbook on pages 39–45. To make teaching easier, use the instruction icons as cues for leading the session. Be sure to insert your facility's policies and procedures whenever appropriate.

2. Encourage participant discussion when appropriate.

3. Hand out the quiz and allow adequate time for each participant to finish.

4. Give certificates of completion to those who correctly answered at least seven of the questions.

Answer key

1. Behavioral	2. Purpose	3. Communication	4. Lighting
5. Diversion	6. False	7. D	8. False
9. Supervision	10. C		

Reasons for wandering and eloping

Wandering usually has a purpose.

It may be a form of communication when language skills are lost. A resident with dementia may be trying to communicate that he or she needs to urinate, or perhaps he or she is hungry or thirsty, or needs to rest. Many things can trigger wandering—loud conversations in the background, noise of kitchen utensils, or a loud TV.

Other reasons for wandering

- If wandering occurs at the same time every day, it may be an old routine that causes it. For instance, if a resident attempts to leave every day at 5 p.m. he may believe he is going home from work. When he sees staff leaving, it reinforces his thought.

- If wandering usually occurs in the late afternoon or evening or during the night, the individual may have Sundowners syndrome. Sundowners is also called nighttime confusion. When it begins to get dark, the person becomes increasingly more confused. The individual may act very anxious, agitated, or angry. This may lead to wandering, pacing the floors, and nervousness. Sometimes people with Sundowners have rapid mood changes, crying or becoming paranoid, aggressive, or even violent. Often they begin looking and calling for family members or try to leave the building.

- Loss of memory.

- Excess energy.

- Discomfort or pain.

- Stress, anxiety, and agitation.

- Being in a new environment.

- Inability to recognize familiar people, places, and objects.

- Restlessness or boredom.

- Trying to express emotions such as fear or loneliness.

- Curiosity.

 THE CNA TRAINING SOLUTION: TRAINER'S MANUAL, SECOND EDITION

- Medication side effects.

- Sight of things that trigger memories—e.g., boots and a coat next to the door may signal it is time to go out.

- Wanting to escape from a noisy or busy place.

- Confusing night and day.

- Fatigue. Residents with dementia tire easily and become restless.

Managing wandering and elopement

Diversion activities may help with wandering or pacing behaviors. These activities can capture the resident's interest and take his or her mind off the feelings that are causing the wandering:

- Hobbies

- Reading

- Social interaction

- Listening to music

- Pet therapy

Provide a platform-style rocking chair that moves back and forth easily but has a stable, immobile base. The more the resident rocks, the more effective this therapy is on easing depression, anxiety, and tension. When someone is upset or restless, offer a rocking chair.

 A resident may be looking for a family member. A memory album, memory box, or photographs of family members on the wall might help.

To minimize restlessness, excess energy, or boredom:

- Provide and encourage regular exercise.

- Wandering may be a way of keeping occupied, so help occupy the person by involving them in a fun activity.

- Let the resident pace where it is safe.

- Are bright lights and noise from the TV or radio adding to the confusion or restlessness?

- A person who has spent a lifetime doing chores may need something to do. Provide purposeful activities, such as folding towels or cleaning.

Residents may wander because they have forgotten where they are, or are having difficulty finding the bathroom or their room.

- Post photographs on the doors to various rooms, including a picture of the resident on the door to his or her room. Use a picture of the resident as a young adult, since that may be more recognizable.

- Use color schemes to identify different areas.

To minimize restlessness and confusion late in the afternoon or evening (Sundowners):

- Keep the resident active in the morning and encourage a rest after lunch.

- A walk outdoors while it is still light outside might reduce restlessness.

- Turn the lights on inside the individual's room or apartment before it gets dark out.

- Take advantage of as much natural light as possible while it is still light outdoors, but before it begins to get dark close the blinds and shades so the person can't see outside.

If the individual tends to wander at about the same time every day, try to find out the person's history. Is she a mother who picked her children up at three o'clock every afternoon? Staff may need to leave by a door that the individual cannot see, so he or she doesn't get the idea that it is time to go.

It is particularly important to watch exit doors when visitors are coming or going. Seeing people leave may make the person with dementia think it is time for him or her to leave also. Slipping out the door behind visitors is a common exit strategy for wanderers.

Creating a safe environment for wandering

If you determine the wandering is not associated with a physical need, such as thirst, hunger, pain, fatigue, or the need to urinate, you might just provide space for walking or exploring. Some facilities make the halls circular so residents won't come to a dead end.

It is not a good idea, however, to let residents pace constantly for long periods of time. Some people with dementia will walk most of the day and sometimes the night, exhausting themselves in the process unless someone stops them. Many sleep for only short periods and walk most of the night, not even stopping to eat. This kind of excessive wandering is harmful, but short periods of walking can work off restlessness if done in a safe setting.

To create a safe environment for wandering at your facility, consider doing the following:

- Remove throw rugs, electrical cords, and other things that might cause a resident to trip or fall.

- Arrange furniture simply and keep public areas uncluttered to provide room for walking. Keep the furniture arrangement consistently the same so the environment stays familiar.

- Night lights may help at night. Ensure adequate lighting at all times.

- Putting a stop sign on an exit door may stop a confused individual from going any further in that direction. Or, a black mat in front of the door will stop some wanderers (it may look like a hole in the ground to them). Some facilities have used murals with paintings of books or furniture on exit doors, so a wanderer thinks the door is part of the wall and does not attempt to leave by that door. If you want to use this strategy, check with the fire marshal to be sure you are not hindering recognition of an exit door in the event of a fire.

- Try changing the feel of doorknobs that the wandering resident might try to turn. Door knob holders made out of felt material, for example, slip on the knob and make it feel different. This has been effective in preventing some wandering residents from opening doors.

- Have residents with a potential for elopement wear an identity bracelet with name, address, and phone number.

- Keep exit doors alarmed and check alarms daily to ensure they are working.

- Consider safety bracelets that sound an alarm if a wanderer succeeds in getting through any exit doorways.

- Use Check-In/Check-Out Logs so staff is aware of who has left the building for authorized or legitimate reasons.

- Change door codes regularly.

- Do regular checks at certain times of the day and night to see if every resident that is supposed to be in the building is present. You can target these checks specifically for residents with an elopement risk if a total building check is not reasonable or desired. Meals can be good times to ensure that confused residents are where they should be.

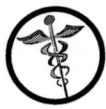

Responding to an elopement

Your facility may have a procedure to follow if someone elopes. Here are the steps to take for an elopement attempt:

1. If you see a resident who you know should not leave trying to exit the building, stop the resident by distracting him or her with something of interest. Offer a diversion activity or a snack to get attention.

2. If that doesn't work and the resident refuses to cooperate, get help from other staff if possible.

3. Whether or not you have help, ***do not leave the resident for any reason.*** A confused person can wander out into the street or fall into a ditch in seconds. Continue redirecting the resident into the building.

Here are the steps that staff should take as soon as you discover that a resident is missing:

1. Conduct a thorough search of the building immediately and rapidly. Organize the search so that you know all areas are covered.

   a. All staff should gather in one place and agree to a plan.

   b. Each employee should have specific instructions for the places he or she is to search. For example, one person might check one side of a hallway while another searches the other side. If the building is a continuous circle or square, have staff members start from opposite directions and meet in the middle.

   c. Look carefully but quickly in every room, every bathroom, every closet, every opening of any type large enough for a person (and remember that people can sometimes fit into very small spaces). Check locked rooms as well.

   d. Look under all beds and in all showers.

2. Do a thorough search of the grounds.

   a. If there is enough help, two people should go outside and walk around the building, each going in the opposite direction and meeting behind the building, then returning inside.

b. One staff member should stay in the residence at all times, so if only two people are working, one will search outside while the other stays with the residents inside. *Be calm* and keep order.

c. If only one person is working, that individual should conduct a quick search of the premises immediately around the building.

d. ***Never*** leave the other residents unattended for more than a few seconds. It may be necessary to go to every exit door and look around immediately outside that door.

e. If you are able to conduct a thorough search of the grounds, do the following, using a flashlight if it is dark outside:

   • Look in every car parked near the building.

   • Check under and behind bushes.

   • Look closely in any bodies of water.

   • Look behind and under rocks and mounds.

   • Look inside any ditches, holes, or hollow areas.

   • Walk around any nearby hill.

   • Look into and under any construction materials or other objects on or near the premises.

3. If you do not find the resident, do the following:

   a. Call the administrator and explain what has happened. Follow his or her instructions.

   b. Depending on your administrator's instructions, you may need to call 911 to notify the police and emergency responders.

   c. Someone will need to contact the resident's responsible family member or other authorized representative. The administrator will probably do this.

   d. The administrator may want you to call the resident's physician.

   e. Only share information with people authorized to receive it.

4. If you do not locate the resident and the police take over, be ready to provide important information about the resident:

   a. Name, nickname, age, and gender

   b. A photograph

   c. Physical description, including height, weight, race, eye and hair color, and color and type of clothing worn (if known)

   d. Time discovered missing and where resident was last seen

   e. Mental and physical condition

   f. Addresses and phone numbers of any known friends and relatives, and previous home address (if known)

When the resident is returned or found

- Do not scold or show anxiety. The resident may be confused and frightened.

- Reassure the resident.

- Get the individual back into a regular routine as soon as possible.

- Contact everyone whom you informed of the elopement, letting them know the resident has been located.

- A nurse or physician should assess the resident as soon as possible.

Documentation

In addition to documenting the elopement in your service notes, whoever discovered the resident missing will need to fill out an incident report. Also complete an incident report if the resident tried to elope but was not successful. In the report, be sure to include the following information:

- The time the resident was last seen, what the staff did, and the facts of how the elopement occurred

- The resident's physical, emotional, and mental status before the elopement

- How, when, and where the resident was found, and the resident's condition when found

- Describe any injuries and what was done to treat the injuries

- Describe the resident's clothing, the temperature outside, and how much and which areas of skin were exposed

- List all the people that were notified of the elopement.

Managing Elopement and Wandering Behaviors

Name: _____

Date: _____   Score: _____

Directions: Fill in the blanks or circle the correct answer.

1. Dementia causes changes in the brain, which in turn cause _____ problems.

2. Wandering usually has a _____.

3. Wandering may be a form of _____ when language skills are lost.

4. To help someone with symptoms of Sundowners syndrome, provide good _____ before it begins to get dark.

5. _____ activities may capture a resident's interest and distract him or her from the feelings that are causing problem behaviors.

6. If you see a resident eloping, you should call for help before doing anything else.
   True   False

7. What is the first thing you should do when you discover a resident is missing?
   a. Write an incident report   c. Call the family
   b. Call the police   d. Conduct a thorough search

8. When you find a resident who has eloped, be sure he or she knows how angry you are and how much trouble he or she has caused.
   True   False

9. Since no facility can be elopement-proof, staff _____ of residents with dementia is essential.

10. If a resident with dementia who usually comes to meals doesn't appear for a meal, it is best to:
    a. Assume the resident is sleeping or not feeling hungry, and leave him or her alone.
    b. Remind yourself to go check on the resident later, when you're not as busy.
    c. Immediately look for the resident.
    d. Call the family.

 Also appears on your CD-ROM.

CERTIFICATE OF COMPLETION

This is to certify that

_____

has read and successfully passed the final exam of

Elopement and wandering

_____

Supervisor name

Mental illness

Overview

This lesson is designed to help workers understand the different types of mental illness.

Program time
Approximately 45 minutes

Learning objectives
After completing this lesson, participants will be able to do the following:

- Recognize symptoms of mental illness

- Describe characteristics of mental illness

- List treatments and care measures for mental illness

Preparation

1. Familiarize yourself with the information by reviewing the lesson prior to teaching it.

2. Print and pass out appropriate handout(s) when instructed.

3. Print out a quiz and certificate for each learner from the CD-ROM.

Method

1. Deliver a mini-lecture covering the material in the workbook on pages 47–52. To make teaching easier, use the instruction icons as cues for leading the session. Be sure to insert your facility's policies and procedures whenever appropriate.

2. Encourage participant discussion when appropriate..

3. Hand out the quiz and allow adequate time for each participant to finish.

4. Give certificates of completion to those who correctly answered at least seven of the questions.

Answer key

1. Brain	6. False	10. Dry mouth, constipation,
2. D	7. Obsessive-compulsive	appetite changes, weight gain,
3. True	8. False	blurred vision, drowsiness,
4. False	9. True	loss of sexual function
5. Depression		11. Mania

Mental illness

Mental health problems are common among the elderly, the chronically ill, and the disabled. Since people with mental illness can demonstrate many different symptoms, we often do not recognize the signs. As a result, many people do not receive the medications or treatments that might help. Caregivers should learn how to recognize mental illness and how to care for the mentally ill.

Mental illness is a brain disorder that causes abnormal ways of *thinking*, *feeling*, or *acting*.

Symptoms of abnormal thinking

- **Delusions.** This means believing things that are not true. A person might think someone wants to kill or hurt him or her.

- **Hallucinations.** This means seeing or hearing things that are not really there. A person who is hallucinating might hear people talking to him or her when no one is.

- **Confused thinking.** The person might be illogical or not understand things happening around him or her.

- **Suicidal thoughts.** Someone with a mental illness might have frequent or constant thoughts of killing him or herself.

Symptoms of abnormal behavior

- Disruptive or antisocial behaviors

- Changes in sleeping routines

- Changes in eating habits

- Alcohol, drug, or medicine abuse

- Very slow or fast speech or movements

- Agitated behavior or fits of temper

- Changes in hygiene practices

- Unwillingness to cooperate

- Easily distracted, can't pay attention

- Withdrawal from normal activities or from people

Symptoms of abnormal feelings

- Frequent mood changes

- Depression or sadness

- Anxiety, worry, or panic

- Irritability or anger

- Frequent crying, tearfulness

- Apathy, poor motivation

- Hopeless and/or helpless feelings

- Excessively low or high self-esteem

- Excessively energetic or euphoric

- Poor judgment, impulsiveness

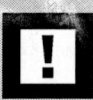 Ask learners to describe some of the characteristics of mentally ill residents and associated care challenges.

Types of mental illness

Many different things cause mental health problems. Sometimes mental disorders are genetic, meaning they run in families. Mental illnesses can be caused by reactions to stressful events, by imbalances in the body's chemistry, or by a combination of several factors. The symptoms of mental illness occur because the brain is not functioning well. This affects the person's thought processes, emotions, and/or behavior.

 It is important to remember that mentally ill people usually cannot control the way they think, feel, or behave. Mental illness is not the person's fault. They cannot help themselves.

The seven main types of mental disorders are: cognitive, dissociative, anxiety, eating, mood, personality, and psychotic disorders.

Cognitive disorders

Cognitive impairment is a loss of mental abilities and awareness that occurs in varying degrees with a variety of underlying causes. In the elderly it is usually caused by physical changes in the brain. Symptoms include loss of intellectual abilities, personality changes, forgetfulness, inability to concentrate, poor judgment, and verbal confusion. It can hinder a person's ability to do daily activities.

- **Dementia.** This disorder involves the parts of the brain that control thought, memory, and language. Healthy brain tissue deteriorates, causing a steady loss in memory and mental abilities. Strokes or changes in the brain's blood supply may result in the death of brain tissue. Symptoms of dementia caused by problems with blood vessels can appear suddenly, whereas symptoms develop slowly in persons with Alzheimer's disease. Although found primarily in the elderly, 50% of people with AIDS develop dementia.

- **Alzheimer's disease.** This is the most common form of dementia among people age 65 and older. It may begin with slight memory loss and confusion, but eventually leads to a severe, permanent mental impairment that destroys the ability to remember, reason, learn, and imagine. On the average, people die within 10 years of getting Alzheimer's.

Dissociative disorders

These disorders come in many forms, all thought to stem from traumatic events. When an extremely stressful event occurs, the person is too overwhelmed to process it and tries to cope with the trauma by separating him or herself from the experience. This can lead to loss of memory or the formation of separate personalities.

- **Dissociative identity disorder.** This disorder is evidenced by two or more personalities or identities that control a person's consciousness at different times. It used to be called multiple personality disorder.

- **Dissociative amnesia.** In this disorder the person forgets some or all of his or her personal information, such as who he or she is or where he or she lives.

Anxiety disorders

Anxiety causes physical symptoms such as rapid shallow breathing, increased heart rate, sweating, and trembling. It can cause emotional symptoms including alarm, dread, and apprehension. Treatment may include medication, therapy, or a combination.

- **Panic disorder.** This is a sudden onset of intense fear, apprehension, and impending doom that may last from minutes to hours. Approximately one in three people with panic disorder develop agoraphobia. Persons with agoraphobia are afraid of having attacks in public, so they avoid leaving the house.

- **Post-traumatic stress disorder.** Persons with this disorder reexperience the anxiety associated with a previous traumatic event. Many times it is caused by exposure to an extremely stressful event, such as abuse or rape.

- **Phobias.** A person with a phobia feels very anxious when exposed to a particular object or situation, such as a high place. The person fears and avoids whatever causes the anxiety.

- **Obsessive-compulsive disorder (OCD).** OCD is characterized by the need to maintain control, order, neatness, cleanliness, and/or perfection. People with OCD feel compelled to perform repetitive acts such as handwashing or repeatedly checking to be sure a door is locked.

- **Generalized anxiety disorder (GAD).** This disorder may occur at any age. It is diagnosed after at least six months of persistent, excessive anxiety and worry.

Personality disorders

Personality disorders are chronic conditions with biological and psychological causes. Psychotherapy is the treatment, sometimes along with medications.

- **Borderline personality disorder.** This disorder is characterized by impulsive behavior, unstable social relationships, and intense anger. These persons can have periods of psychotic thinking, paranoia, and hallucinations.

- **Obsessive-compulsive personality.** These people tend to be high achievers. They are dependable and orderly but can't adjust to change and are intolerant of mistakes. They can be uncomfortable with relationships. This is not the same as obsessive-compulsive disorder.

- **Passive-aggressive personality.** These people hide hostile feelings and try to control or punish others.

- **Narcissistic personality.** Persons with this personality feel superior to others and expect to be admired. They are seen as self-centered and arrogant.

- **Antisocial personality, formerly called psychopathic or sociopathic personality.** These people show no regard for the rights and feelings of others. They do not tolerate frustration and become hostile or violent. They show no remorse or guilt and blame others for their behavior.

Mood disorders

Mood disorders usually involve chemical imbalances in the brain, and are often treated with antidepressants and/or psychotherapy.

- **Depression.** Depression causes severe, prolonged sadness. It can affect a person's thoughts, feelings, behavior, and physical health. It may develop at any age. Depressed people often look sad or expressionless and lose interest in normal activities. Depression is the leading cause of disability in the United States, affecting more women than men.

 Older people often think sadness is part of aging, or that forgetfulness, loss of appetite, and insomnia are symptoms of dementia. Depression is not a sign of old age. It is an illness and needs treatment like any other illness.

- **Bipolar disorder,** also called manic depression, causes episodes of severe mania (euphoria, increased energy and confidence) and depression (sadness, fatigue, poor concentration) that alternate with periods of normal mood. It occurs equally in men and women.

- **Seasonal affective disorder (SAD).** This disorder is characterized by recurrent bouts of depression in certain months of the year, usually fall and winter. Symptoms include oversleeping, carbohydrate craving, weight gain, lethargy, and social withdrawal. SAD is treated by bright fluorescent light, which alters the levels of brain chemicals.

Psychotic disorders

In acute phases of psychosis a person loses touch with reality and is unable to meet the ordinary demands of life. Most psychotic episodes are brief.

- **Schizophrenia.** Schizophrenia is a severe and chronic brain disorder that impairs the ability to think clearly, make decisions, and relate to others. Persons with this disorder suffer frightening symptoms that leave them fearful and withdrawn. One out of every hundred people has this treatable illness, men and women alike. It involves problems with brain structure and chemistry. People with schizophrenia do not have a "split personality." They may have delusions or hallucinations. They cannot tell what is real and what is not real. People with this disorder may talk to themselves, walk in circles, pace, and have difficulty carrying on conversations. There may be a lack of facial expression. They may be unable to follow through with activities they start.

Treatment of mental illnesses

Mental health disorders are treatable, and many people recover. Medications, psychotherapy, psychoeducation, electroconvulsive therapy, and self-help and support groups are used in the treatment of mental illnesses. Anything that improves a person's quality of life can help, such as pets, social events, activities, or reality orientation classes. Many communities and facilities are affiliated with mental health professionals that can screen for mental health problems and conduct therapy sessions.

Medications

Many of the medicines used to treat mental illness cause unpleasant side effects. Some of the more common ones are dry mouth, constipation, blurred vision, appetite changes, loss of sexual function, drowsiness, and weight gain.

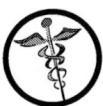

Drinking eight glasses of water a day and eating fruits and vegetables can help with some of this.

Antipsychotic drugs can cause tremors, stiffness, muscle contraction and rigidity, restlessness, and loss of facial expression. Elderly people and those that have taken these medicines for years sometimes develop a condition called tardive dyskinesia. This causes uncontrolled facial movements and jerking or twisting movements of other body parts. This condition can be treated with medication.

Psychotherapy

Psychotherapy is the use of psychological techniques to change behaviors, feelings, thoughts, or habits. It is recommended for persons experiencing emotional distress.

- **Behavior management.** The aim of behavior management is to increase the occurrence of desirable behavior by rewarding the person for acting correctly. Unsuitable behavior is reduced by giving negative consequences.

- **Cognitive therapy.** Cognitive therapy emphasizes a rational and positive view. This therapy attempts to change destructive thought patterns that can lead to disappointment and frustration. It is effective with anxiety and depression.

- **Psychoeducation.** Psychoeducation is teaching people about their illness, treatment, and how to recognize a relapse. Teaching coping skills to the family will help them deal with an ill relative.

- **Self-help and support groups.** These groups help because members give each other ongoing support. It's comforting to know others have the same or similar problems. These groups can also help families work together for needed research, treatments, and community programs.

Mental Illness

QUIZ

Name: _____

Date: _____   **Score:** _____

Directions: Write the correct answer in the blank or circle the correct answer.

1. **Mental illnesses are disorders of the** _____.

2. **Mental illnesses may be caused by:**
    a. Genetic factors   b. Chemical imbalances   c. Reactions to stressful events   d. All of the above

3. **Anxiety may cause physical symptoms as well as emotional symptoms.**
    True   False

4. **Post-traumatic stress syndrome is caused by overreacting to something mildly unpleasant.**
    True   False

5. **The leading cause of disability in the U.S. is** _____.

6. **Depression is a normal part of getting older.**
    True   False

7. **If a person must have everything in order and in its place and is continually cleaning, you might suspect they have** _____ _____ **disorder.**

8. **A person with schizophrenia has a "split personality."**
    True   False

9. **A person with schizophrenia may hear or see things that are not real.**
    True   False

10. **Some of the common side effects of medications that treat mental illness are:**
    _____

11. **A person with bipolar disorder has mood swings from severe** _____ **to depression.**

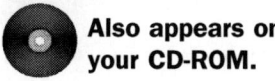

Also appears on your CD-ROM.

CERTIFICATE OF COMPLETION

This is to certify that

_____

has read and successfully passed the final exam of

Mental illness

_____
Supervisor name

Communication guidelines

Overview

Today you will teach staff how to communicate effectively with residents.

Program time
Approximately 30 minutes

Learning objectives
After completing this lesson, participants will be able to do the following:

- State the meaning of communication

- Demonstrate how to be an active listener

- Demonstrate how to speak effectively

- List nonverbal ways of communicating

- List the five don'ts of communication

- Explain how to communicate in difficult situatiions

Preparation

1. Familiarize yourself with the information by reviewing the lesson prior to teaching it.

2. Print and pass out appropriate handout(s) when instructed.

3. Print out a quiz and certificate for each learner from the CD-ROM.

Method

1. Deliver a mini-lecture covering the material in the workbook on pages 53–57.

2. Encourage participant discussion when appropriate, and ask for additional ideas to help residents deal with the effects of aging.

3. Hand out the quiz and allow adequate time for each participant to finish.

4. Give certificates of completion to those who correctly answered at least seven of the questions.

Answer key

1. D	2. D	3. B	4. C
5. A	6. D	7. B	8. C

9. Offer opinions, become defensive, make judgments, ask why, give empty assurances
10. A

How communication works

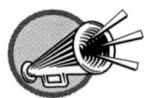
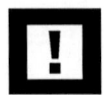

All of us are communicating all of the time. As I speak these words to you, I am sending messages to you with my voice, my facial expressions, my posture, and my hand motions. Even the way I am dressed communicates something. You are also communicating with me and with each other. By the looks on your faces and your body language, you tell me whether you are bored or interested. You communicate with me through words, but also by your dress and the way you do your job.

We communicate with our residents in all these ways too, and we should be alert to what they are telling us through the various ways they try to communicate with us. For communication to occur, someone must send a message and someone must receive it. If a message is not received and understood, we are not communicating. To be a good communicator, we must learn how to find out whether our messages are received. We must learn how to ask questions and listen to feedback from our residents.

Many things can hinder good communication. Eyesight and hearing problems, illness, stress, medications, emotions, fatigue, confusion, language or cultural differences, and even personality differences are some of the things that might a effect how well a message is delivered and received. Learning how to communicate effectively can go a long way toward helping our residents feel happy and secure.

 Learning activity

Ask learners to work in pairs and take turns telling their partners about someone who is important to them, such as a child. After each learner finishes, his or her partner should rate whether the speech was effective, based on the six points outlined in "Effective talking." The learner who did the speaking should rate his or her partner based on the ten points outlined in "Active listening." After everyone has had a turn, ask learners to share what they learned.

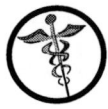

Active listening

To communicate well, learn to listen well. Practice these listening skills:

1. Make eye contact.

2. Sit at eye level.

3. Look relaxed and interested.

4. Avoid making distracting movements.

5. Lean toward the talker in "listening posture."

6. Nod your head or make other understanding gestures.

7. Make sounds of understanding and interest, such as "hmmm" or "oh my," at appropriate times.

8. Ask questions about what the speaker is saying, to clarify a point, focus the conversation, and show interest.

9. Touch the speaker or hold his or her hand if appropriate.

10. Use the Seven Skills of Active Listening.

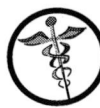

Effective talking

Practice these skills to help get your message across:

1. Speak clearly and distinctly.

2. Use simple words and sentences.

3. Give all the information the person needs, such as who you are and what you are going to do.

4. Use descriptive gestures to reinforce your words.

5. Use humor when appropriate.

6. Use expressions, gestures, and body language to reinforce your message.

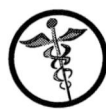 ## The five don'ts of communication

Try to eliminate these communication methods. They are ineffective and prevent good communication from happening.

1. **Don't offer your opinions.** Help your residents make their own decisions. Don't tell them what you think they should or shouldn't do.

2. **Don't become defensive.** When a resident criticizes you or someone else, reflect his or her concern back to him or her so you can learn more about the problem.

3. **Don't make judgments.** Instead of showing disapproval, ask the resident about his or her reasons for acting or feeling a certain way. Be open to differences of opinion.

4. **Don't ask "why."** "Why" questions make people feel more defensive. Word questions in a nonthreatening way, such as asking calmly, "What happened?" or "Can you tell me about it?"

5. **Don't give empty assurances.** "Everything's going to be fine" isn't necessarily true. Focus on helping the resident talk about his or her concerns.

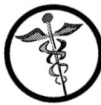 ## Seven skills of active listening

Use these skills to become a better listener:

1. Use small encouraging sounds (such as "uh-huh") and nod your head. Don't appear impatient or hurried.

2. Be other-focused. Ask questions so others will want to talk about themselves. Focus conversations on the person you are talking to, not yourself.

3. Reflect. Keep conversations focused on the other person by reflecting back their thoughts and feelings. Concentrate on their feelings and concerns.

4. Be quiet. Give the speaker plenty of time to collect his or her thoughts and share his or her feelings.

5. Clarify. Find out exactly what someone means when he or she says something. You can learn valuable information this way. Clarify anything that raises a question in your mind.

6. Ask open questions. Ask questions that require more than just a "yes" or "no" answer. You get more information that way.

7. Repeat. To be sure you understand something, repeat what you hear in your own words, then ask if you repeated it correctly.

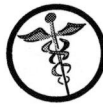

Dealing with an angry person

1. Keep your mood, facial expression, body language, and voice calm, quiet, and relaxed.

2. Do not argue. This will only increase the individual's anger and cause the incident to get worse.

3. Maintain eye contact.

4. Keep a clear exit for yourself, making sure the angry person doesn't block your way to the doorway.

5. Use the skill of reflection. Reflect his or her feelings back to the angry person to get a sense of what is bothering him or her.

6. Don't pass judgment on someone's words or behavior. Stay open minded and listen actively to hear the underlying feelings and concerns.

7. After you have listened to the reasons for the person's anger, help him or her solve the problem or handle the situation.

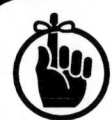 If these tactics don't work or you fear harm, call for help and notify your supervisor immediately.

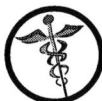

How to communicate with residents who have speaking, hearing, or understanding problems

1. Allow plenty of time for the person to respond to something you say.

2. Turn off or remove distractions such as a television or radio. You might have to close the door to the room if there is noise in the hallway.

3. Stay on the resident's "good" side, where his or her hearing or speech is best. Let him or her see your mouth as you speak.

4. Don't rush the person or finish sentences for him or her unless you can help by patiently supplying a word or two.

5. When you are speaking, use the correct voice volume. You may have to be louder if the person is hard of hearing; however, remember that individuals with dementia or people who have had a stroke aren't necessarily hard of hearing. A normal volume works best in these situations.

6. Use short, simple words and phrases.

7. When the person has difficulty finding the right words, ask him or her to point to words on a board or a piece of paper. Encourage residents to use gestures such as head nodding and hand motions.

8. When giving directions, state one instruction at a time. Break down your directions into simple steps.

Either in their workbooks or with a partner, have learners break down a task (like face washing) into short, simple directions.

QUIZ

Communication guidelines

Name: _____

Date: _____   Score: _____

Circle one correct answer for each question.

1. **Which of the following statements use the listening skill of reflection?**
   a. You seem worried about something.
   b. What do you think is the best thing to do?
   c. So you think it might be hard to follow the doctor's orders?
   d. All of the above.

2. **If a resident is having difficulty saying the right words, you should:**
   a. Be silent and allow time for the resident to think.
   b. Provide words or pictures on a board or paper for the resident to point to.
   c. Guess at what he is trying to say.
   d. Both A and B.

3. **Open-ended questions are good for obtaining information, but it is better to ask questions that can be answered with a yes or no if:**
   a. You are in a hurry.
   b. The resident has difficulty speaking.
   c. The resident has difficulty hearing.
   d. You don't want too much information

4. **Communication only occurs when:**
   a. Someone is talking.
   b. Someone is listening.
   c. A message is both given and received.
   d. The message is written down.

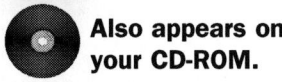 **Also appears on your CD-ROM.**

QUIZ

Communication guidelines (cont.)

5. **Nonverbal communication occurs through:**
   a. Gestures, expressions, posture, and dress.
   b. Silence.
   c. Speech.
   d. None of the above.

6. **If a resident says something that raises a question in your mind, you should:**
   a. Ignore it.
   b. Tell him he's thinking the wrong way.
   c. Offer your opinion.
   d. Clarify by asking the resident what he means.

7. **When a resident is angry, you should:**
   a. Give him a hug.
   b. Remain calm and ask what is wrong.
   c. Argue with him.
   d. Stay away.

8. **When speaking, it is important to:**
   a. Rush through your thoughts
   b. Speak loudly.
   c. Speak clearly and use simple words and phrases.
   d. Avoid looking directly at anyone.

9. **List the five donts"of communication. (5 pts.) Don't:**

   _____   _____   _____
   _____   _____

10. **It is best if our conversations with residents focus on:**
    a. The resident
    b. Other people
    c. Ourselves
    d. The facility

CERTIFICATE OF COMPLETION

This is to certify that

_____

has read and successfully passed the final exam of

Communication guidelines

_____
Supervisor name

Coping with death

Overview

Today you will teach staff how cope with death and how to help others cope.

Program time
Approximately 30 minutes

Learning objectives
After completing this lesson, participants will be able to do the following:

- Describe grief and its spiritual, emotional, and physical effects

- Recognize the symptoms of grief in themselves, coworkers, residents, and families

- Learn to verbalize feelings and listen to others

- Apply means of dealing with grief following the death of a resident

Preparation

1. Familiarize yourself with the information by reviewing the lesson prior to teaching it.

2. Print and pass out appropriate handout(s) when instructed.

3. Print out a quiz and certificate for each learner from the CD-ROM.

Method

1. Deliver a mini-lecture covering the material in the workbook on pages 59–64.

2. Encourage participant discussion when appropriate, and ask for additional ideas to help in coping with death.

3. Hand out the quiz and allow adequate time for each participant to finish.

4. Give certificates of completion to those who correctly answered at least seven of the questions.

Answer key

1. Death, job, divorce, health (choose 3)	5. True	8. Spiritually, emotionally,
2. Sadness, anger, guilt	6. False	behaviorally, physically
3. All but C	7. False	9. False
4. Coworkers		10. True

Introduction

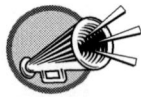

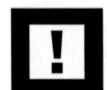

When a resident dies, all of a professional caregiver's energies go into helping the family and other residents cope with the loss of their loved one. We often forget that caregivers also grieve over the loss of people they care about. Caregiving workers develop relationships and attachments with residents, so when a resident dies, workers may experience grief, even though they do not always recognize it.

Although we cannot avoid it, this exposure to suffering and death is very stressful for the caregiver. Usually there is no opportunity to grieve, and over time it takes a toll. Many times we must cope with difficult feelings without help.

The sudden death of a resident who appears to be doing well is particularly difficult to handle. A range of emotions arise from this event: intense shock and grief, feelings of confusion and helplessness, and even guilt that the death was somehow the result of something that was overlooked or preventable.

Family members often react to the death of a loved one with anger and frustration. They want answers and are not always polite; they may even be abusive at times. On the other hand, if the staff has had the resident for a while and has gotten to know the family, there is usually more trust and the family does not hold the staff responsible for the death—but they may lean heavily on the staff for comfort and support.

It is important for caregiving workers to find some way of coping with the range of emotions and issues that accompany death—whether it is a good cry or a regular grief session with coworkers. Facing suffering, disability, and death day after day at the workplace causes increasing stress and drains the energy of the care provider. Learning how to manage difficult emotions helps us in many ways. Our lives are less stressful when we know how to deal with guilt, anger, anxiety, and sadness.

 Death is a part of life. Death gives meaning to our existence by reminding us how precious life is.

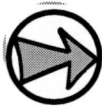

Ask participants to think about personal experiences they have had with grief. If any are willing, give them time to talk about their experience. Encourage them to discuss the things and people that helped them work through their grief.

What is grief?

- Grief is a reaction to any loss—death of a loved one, divorce, loss of health, loss of a job.

- We express grief through feelings such as anger, guilt, sadness, or loneliness. Grief creates a state of disharmony.

- Grief affects people spiritually, emotionally, behaviorally, and physically:

  - **Spiritually:** Grief affects spiritual convictions. A person may feel angry at God or question beliefs.

  - **Emotionally:** A person may experience rapid mood swings or bouts of anger, crying, or irritability. He or she may become depressed.

  - **Behaviorally:** A person who is experiencing difficult emotions usually acts out those emotions in behavior, such as being tearful, short-tempered, irritable, anxious, withdrawn, or unable to function normally.

  - **Physically:** A person may lose his or her appetite, have stomach or head pain, feel exhausted, have trouble sleeping, or not function well.

What do we feel when a resident dies?

After the death of someone we care about, we experience bereavement, which means "to be deprived by death." When a death takes place, most people experience a wide range of emotions. These feelings are normal reactions to loss. Sometimes the intensity and duration of the emotions or the swift mood changes catch us by surprise, making us think we're going crazy. These feelings, however, are healthy and appropriate and help us come to terms with loss. The loss of someone we care about is life's most stressful event and can cause a major emotional crisis.

These are some of the emotions we can expect:

- **Shock, denial, disbelief, and confusion.** These reactions are part of the emotional numbness often felt when death occurs. Our first thought may be, "No, it can't be!"

- **Depression.** Unresolved grief can cause long-term sadness.

- **Guilt.** Some blame themselves, wondering if they could have done more.

- **Anger.** We sometimes blame others for a death. We ask, "What if the doctor had done this or that?"

- **Anxiety.** We might feel nervous or worried or feel that we are not in control.

- **Yearning.** We may desperately long for the person to come back.

- **Apathy or despair.** We may feel hopeless and think no one understands how we feel or that everything is pointless. Life may lose its meaning.

- **Acceptance.** Slowly, we learn to cope with death.

Not every person will experience all these emotions, and the emotions will not occur in any particular order. It takes time to fully absorb the impact of a loss.

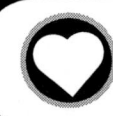

Unresolved grief can lead to feelings of anxiety and depression.

Mourning

Mourning is the natural process we go through to accept a loss. Mourning may include religious traditions honoring the dead or gathering with friends and family. Mourning is personal and may last years.

It is very important to allow people to express these feelings. Often we avoid, ignore, or deny the existence of death. At first it may seem helpful to separate ourselves from the pain, but we cannot avoid grieving forever. Someday those feelings will need to be resolved or they may cause physical or emotional illness.

Reactions to death are influenced by the circumstances and by the relationship with the person who died.

A child's death arouses an overwhelming sense of injustice—for lost potential, unfulfilled dreams, and senseless suffering. Parents may feel responsible for the child's death, no matter how irrational that may seem.

A spouse's death is very traumatic. In addition to the severe emotional shock, the death may cause a financial or caregiving crisis and may necessitate major social adjustments.

Elderly people may be especially vulnerable when they lose a spouse because it means losing a lifetime of shared experiences. Feelings of loneliness may be compounded by the deaths of close friends.

How can we cope and help others cope?

When we learn how to manage our emotions, we are better able to cope with a resident's death and help friends and family. We also help ourselves stay healthy, since unresolved guilt, anger, anxiety, and sadness can cause illness.

Managing guilt

When we feel guilty, we blame ourselves for doing something we think we shouldn't have done or for not doing something we think we should have done. We compare ourselves to an ideal picture of who we wish we were and feel guilty when we don't live up to this.

If you are feeling unrealistic expectations and false guilt, the best thing to do is to recognize it and shut it down. When you feel guilty, tell yourself the guilt is unreasonable and unproductive. Be firm with yourself!

Managing anger

We feel angry when life does not meet our expectations. We may be angry that we have lost someone important to us. To manage anger, ask:

- Are your expectations realistic?

- Is your anger justified?

If you feel your anger is justified, talk about it with someone you trust. That person may be able to help you see and understand things in a different light. When you talk about it, take responsibility for your anger. Say, "I feel angry about this because I expected the doctor to help this person get well."

We must let go of unrealistic expectations of ourselves and of others. We should learn to plan around things we cannot change.

Managing anxiety

Feeling anxious is a normal everyday emotion, but it can be magnified by thinking, "I can't handle this" or fearing that you won't be able to deal with something. We make our anxieties worse when we doubt our ability to cope.

Relaxation techniques are helpful for managing anxiety. These techniques involve:

- Deep breathing, using stomach muscles to pull air in

- Progressive tensing and relaxation of muscles, concentrating on one muscle at a time

- Meditation and prayer

- Hot bath or shower

- Cup of hot tea

- Exercising

- Visualizing peaceful scenes

Living with grief

There are many ways to cope effectively with grief:

- **Seek out caring people.** Find friends who can understand your feelings.

- **Express your feelings.** Tell others how you are feeling.

- **Be patient.** It can take months or even years to absorb a loss.

- **Take care of your health.** Eat well and get plenty of rest. Don't depend on medication or alcohol to deal with your grief.

- **Postpone major life changes.** Wait a while before making any major changes, such as changing jobs. You should give yourself time to adjust.

- **Seek outside help when necessary.** If your grief seems like it is too much to bear, seek professional assistance.

 ## Giving support to others

The best way to promote healing when someone is grieving is to listen. We express feelings through spoken words, so listening helps the grief-stricken person express, examine, and understand their emotions. Crying with someone can be healthy and healing, if done at an appropriate time and place. While each person hurts individually, we can grieve together and support each other.

To support someone who is grieving, do the following:

- **Share the sorrow.** Allow them—even encourage them—to talk about their feelings of loss and share memories of the deceased.

- **Don't offer false comfort.** It doesn't help the grieving person to say, "It was for the best," or "You'll get over it in time." Instead, offer a simple expression of sorrow and take time to listen.

- **Offer practical help.** Give needed recourses to the grieving person and help him or her make arrangements.

- **Be patient.** Remember that it can take a long time to recover from a major loss. Like any wound, it takes time for grief to heal.

- **Encourage professional help when necessary.** Suggest professional help when you feel someone is experiencing too much pain to cope alone.

Exercise: Helping residents deal with grief

Describe the two following scenarios and ask participants to think of at least three things they could do or say to help the people in these circumstances deal with grief. Learners can write their ideas in their workbooks and then share them with the rest of the class.

Take a look at the following two scenarios. For each, write down three ways you could help the people in these scenarios cope with grief.

1. A resident has just received the news that his only child died in a car accident.

2. A resident who you have taken care of for a long time has passed away unexpectedly. Everyone who has helped this resident with her care is very sad about her death.

Q U I Z

Coping with death

Name: _____

Date: _____   **Score:** _____

Write or circle the correct answer.

1. **List three losses that may cause grief:** _____,
    _____, and _____.

2. **People express grief through feelings of: (list three)** _____,
    _____, and _____.

3. **Some ways to handle anxiety include: (Choose all the correct answers)**
    a. Cup of hot tea   d. Meditation and prayer
    b. Hot bath   e. Exercise
    c. Kicking the furniture   f. Deep breathing

4. **When dealing with grief over a resident's death, the most important thing one can do is talk with** _____.

5. **All caregivers are at risk of grief when someone they have cared for dies.**
    True   False

6. **When you feel sad or angry after a resident's death, you can ignore those feelings and they will go away in time.**
    True   False

7. **Everyone experiences the same emotions and timing when grieving.**
    True   False

8. **Name four ways grief can affect a person:** _____, _____,
    _____, and _____.

9. **Facing suffering, disability, and death day after day makes a caregiver better able to handle stress.**
    True   False

10. **Professional caregivers sometimes do not recognize grief when they experience it.**
    True   False

Also appears on your CD-ROM.

CERTIFICATE OF COMPLETION

This is to certify that

_____

has read and successfully passed the final exam of

Coping with death

_____

Supervisor name